The Organization of Medical Practice and the Practice of Medicine

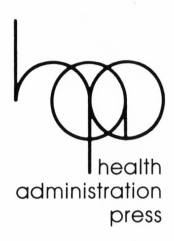

health
administration
press

The Organization of Medical Practice and the Practice of Medicine

Fredric D. Wolinsky

William D. Marder

HEALTH ADMINISTRATION PRESS
ANN ARBOR, MICHIGAN
1985

Library of Congress Cataloging in Publication Data
Wolinsky, Fredric D.
    The organization of medical practice and the practice of medicine.

    Includes bibliographies.
    1. Medicine—Practice. 2. Medical care—Evaluation.
I. Marder, William D. II. Title. [DNLM: 1. Practice
Management, Medical. W 80 W861o]
R728.W64   1985   610'.68   85-7634
ISBN 0-910701-07-5

Health Administration Press
School of Public Health
The University of Michigan
1021 East Huron Street
Ann Arbor, Michigan 48109
(313) 764-1380

For Sally

F. D. W.
College Station, Texas

For Donna, Jessica, and Andrew

W. D. M.
Chicago, Illinois

Contents

Acknowledgments

No book can fail to reflect either the intellectual tradition from which it sprang or the institutional climate in which it grew. This book is no exception to that rule. From the very beginning, the *Profession of Medicine* has played a most important role in the development of research on the relationship between the organization of medical practice and the practice of medicine. For that enormously rich intellectual heritage, we and our fellow health service researchers shall forever be indebted to Professor Eliot Freidson. His remarkable insights have served to spark our interest in how the organization of medical practice affects the practice of medicine. His exacting scholarship remains the classic role model for all those who pursue this issue. We hope that we have met those high standards.

The research reported in this book began, took shape, and came to fruition at the Center for Health Policy Research of the American Medical Association. Several individuals there have been most supportive of our research. In particular, Lynn Jensen fostered a research environment that encouraged our efforts. Lou Goodman and Doug Hough provided departmental resources that facilitated our research. Barbara Corry served as a remarkably efficient research assistant. Without their support and encouragement, our study could never have been completed. For this we are most grateful.

The writing of this book was done primarily at the Center for Health Services Education and Research of St. Louis University Medical Center. Two individuals there were especially supportive. Thomas Dolan provided an environment in which scholarship could flourish. Maxine Lax patiently transcribed the dictated drafts and then proceeded to make all of our editorial revisions with remarkable skill and accuracy. We can not thank these individuals nearly enough.

Although the theory, general analytic model, results, and conclusions reached in this book are new, they are clearly built upon a number of our previous papers.

For permission to use bits, pieces, and themes from our earlier works, we are especially grateful to the editors and publishers of the following journals: the *American Journal of Public Health*, *Health Services Research*, *Medical Care*, the *Milbank Memorial Fund Quarterly*, *Medical Group Management*, and *Profile of Medical Practice 1981*.

Several colleagues read this manuscript and freely offered their comments and suggestions. To Rodney M. Coe and two anonymous referees we express our gratitude and appreciation for helping to clarify our arguments. To Jerry Gaston we extend our special thanks for the extraordinarily detailed and insightful comments on the entire manuscript. Our work has benefited greatly from the help of these very special colleagues.

Finally, we would be remiss not to acknowledge Daphne Grew, Director of Publications, Gene Regenstreif, Executive Editor, and the entire editorial board of the Health Administration Press for their assistance with and continued confidence in our work. From the very first day, their only concern has been with the ultimate publication of a sound, scholarly book. At least for us, this experience has been a pleasant one.

Although we have been very ably assisted in a variety of ways with the research, writing, and production of this book, we alone are responsible for its contents. The views and opinions expressed in this book do not necessarily represent the official position or policy of any of the above named institutions or individuals.

FREDRIC D. WOLINSKY
WILLIAM D. MARDER

November 1984

1

The Conceptual Model of the Organization of Medical Practice: Bringing Freidson's Paradigm into the 1980s

Overview

Our purpose in this monograph is to study the effect of the organization of medical practice on the practice of medicine. We had two motives for exploring this issue. First, there is a general interest among sociologists and economists to investigate whether or not variations in organizational structure affect work outcomes. Sociologists, on the one hand, have traditionally been more concerned with how different organizational structures constrain individuals' attitudes, beliefs, and work patterns. Economists, on the other hand, have traditionally been more concerned with how different organizational structures (i.e., differently configured firms) are related to different levels of productivity. Throughout this monograph we will try to blend those two variations on the same theme into one systematic assessment.

Our second motive is the changing nature of medicine in the United States. To many, especially the general public, it seems as if the American health care delivery system is in a period of remarkable change. The general practice solo physician is no longer the norm. Employee contributions to health insurance premiums are no longer a straightforward federal income tax deduction; indeed, employer contributions to health insurance may soon be treated as taxable income. Cost-plus reimbursement has given way to cost reimbursement, which has given way to cost-minus reimbursement, which is now giving way to prospective payment systems. Health care costs have reached record levels in terms of absolute expenditures, relative expenditures, and the portion of the gross national product spent on health care. And yet, with all of these changes occurring in the health care delivery system, there is no consensus that the health of Americans is as good as it ought to be (see Levine, Feldman and Elinson 1983), even though it may be better than it has ever been (see the Surgeon General's Report 1979).

Accordingly, there is a growing pragmatic desire to identify those organizational structures in which medicine may be practiced as efficiently and effectively as possible. Thus, our examination of the relationship between the organization of medical practice and the practice of medicine has been motivated by and focuses on both theoretical and practical issues.

The purpose of this chapter, then, is to identify the problem at hand, place it in its intellectual and practical context, review relevant previous studies, and show how we intend to attack the problem in order to contribute toward an understanding of the situation. To accomplish this, the remainder of chapter 1 is divided into six sections. First, we review Freidson's (1970) theory on the organization of medical practice. Second, we see how well Freidson's theory corresponds to the subsequent empirical literature. Third, we review the available evidence on the self-selection issue. Fourth, we discuss the emergence of health maintenance organizations and their impact on the organization of medical practice by reviewing both the "promise" and "performance" of HMOs. Fifth, we theoretically disaggregate the incentive bundles that operate in HMOs and discuss the rather thorny issues involved in assessing HMO performance. Finally, we focus on the remaining issues and present the general analytic model that guides our research.

Freidson's Theory of the Organization of Medical Practice

In 1970 Eliot Freidson published an important volume entitled the *Profession of Medicine.* In that book Freidson addresses most of the issues now under discussion in the social science and health disciplines. These issues are organized into four parts, including the formal organization of a profession, the organization of professional performance, the social construction of illness, and consulting professions in a free society. Our primary concern is with part two, which focuses on the organization of professional performance.

Freidson opens his discussion with the following quotation from Karl Mannheim: "Both motives and actions very often originate not from within but from the situation in which individuals find themselves." In this relatively benign fashion, Freidson begins his discussion of one of the classical debates of all times: nature versus nurture. On the one hand, Freidson reminds us that religionists, educationists, and psychologists generally take the nature view, which assumes that the kind of person an individual is determines how he or she will behave, independent of the particular environment. Recast in Freudian terms, this approach believes that the child is the father of the man. On the other hand, Freidson points out that sociologists and economists take the opposite view, which states that an individual's behavior is more a function of environmental pressures, that the environment determines consciousness, and that individuals will behave independently of the kind of person that they are.

To be sure, neither approach is absolutely correct, and Freidson readily recognizes this. He emphasizes, however, that the view one basically accepts greatly influences one's approach to the issue of how medicine is practiced. In particular, Freidson (1970, 88) laments that

> far too much attention has been paid to the personal characteristics and attitudes of individual members of occupations and far too little to the work-settings. This is particularly the case for the professions.

As a result, most efforts to change the behavior of professionals have tried to reform professional curricula rather than modify the circumstances and/or settings in which professionals work.

While Freidson (1970, 89) does not completely ignore the possible effects of such educational socialization, he argues:

> There is some very persuasive evidence that "socialization" does not explain some important elements of professional performance half so well as does the organization of the immediate work environment.

Indeed, after reviewing numerous studies, Freidson (1970, 90) concludes that they

> reinforce my belief that it is at once attractively parsimonious and adequately true to assume that a significant amount of behavior is situational in character—that people are constantly responding to the organized pressures of the situations they are in at any particular time, that what they are is not completely but *more* their present than their past, and that what they do is *more* an outcome of pressures of the situation that they are in than of what they have earlier "internalized."

With that statement, Freidson concludes his justification for the study of the effect of organizational structure on professional performance.

Freidson then begins his analysis of the settings in which medicine is practiced, with an eye toward understanding the major sources of variation in the practice of medicine. Concentrating on the everyday office practice settings, because that is where most medical care takes place, Freidson conceptualizes and describes the four empirical types of practice organization facing physicians during the early 1970s. The four types he describes are the solo practice, association, partnership, and group practice. In describing these practice settings, Freidson recognizes that there are enormous variations within the settings as well as across them and that his intent is to make "some sense out of the variations" by describing the archetypical nature of each of the four settings.

Before proceeding, Freidson carefully points out that, unlike the performance of work by any other professional, the practice of everyday medicine occurs in private. Indeed, Freidson (1970, 91) contrasts this with the work of the other established professions. Their work goes on in the publicity of the court, the church, and the lecture hall as often as in the office. The work of the doctors is characteristically conducted in the closed consulting room or the bedroom. Furthermore, the physician renders personal services to individuals rather than congregations or classes.

Accordingly, while there are different settings in which medicine may be practiced, the practice of medicine in all of these settings fundamentally occurs in private. There is, however, considerable variation in the access to information on how medicine is practiced across the various practice settings. That is, the way medicine is practiced in the privacy of the consulting room is more likely to be known within professional circles in some practice settings than in others.

The most typical form of medical practice in the United States at the time that Freidson wrote the *Profession of Medicine* was solo practice. Freidson (1970, 91) describes solo practice as

a man working by himself in an office in which he secures and equips with his own capital, with patients who have freely chosen him as their personal physician and for whom he assumes responsibility. Stereotypically he lacks any formal connection with colleagues.

According to Freidson, however, solo practice is inherently unstable because the solo physician becomes either severely patient or colleague dependent, depending on whether he or she is in general or family practice or in a medical specialty or subspecialty.

It is the general or family solo practitioners who become client dependent, because without clients their practices would fall apart. In addition, general or family practitioners are not usually the recipients of clients from the referral system; rather, they refer clients to specialists when their services are needed. It is the specialist solo practitioners who become colleague dependent, because they rely on referrals from other specialists or general practitioners for their clients. The ideal referral system among general practitioners (GPs) and specialists (SPs) who are in solo practice is portrayed in figure 1.1, where the different dependencies of the general (i.e., patient dependency) and specialist (i.e., colleague dependency) practitioners are evident.

It would appear, then, that general solo practitioners operate in an independent and unobserved fashion with regard to their colleagues. Thus, it is increasingly difficult to assemble any information indicating poor performance by the solo general practice physician, and the power of informal negative sanctions that might be used to alter the physician's performance is drastically reduced. This is because of the limited interaction and referrals made with the offending solo practice general practitioner. The solo practice specialist, however, is in a much different situation. That specialist is constantly interacting with colleagues and, being dependent on them, permits performance information to be more readily available and allows informal negative sanctions to be more effective.

Figure 1.1   The ideal referral system and dependencies among general
practitioners (GPs) and specialists (SPs) in solo practice

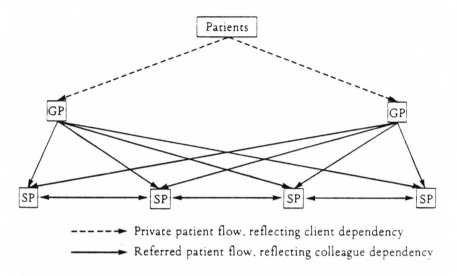

- - - - → Private patient flow, reflecting client dependency

———→ Referred patient flow, reflecting colleague dependency

Source: F. D. Wolinsky, *The Sociology of Health: Principles, Professions, and Issues.* Boston: Little, Brown, 1980. Reprinted with permission.

The issues, however, are not so simple. A discussion of the decision-making process involved with the treatment of one patient by one primary care physician, as shown in figure 1.2, should clarify this (Shortell 1972). In figure 1.2, the patient comes to the primary care physician, who must first decide whether he or she can personally treat the patient. If so, there is no referral to a specialist. If not, a referral takes place, and the total autonomy of the solo primary care physician becomes subject to peer review. Note from figure 1.2 that whether the referral is to a physician specialist, a hospital, or a health agency other than a hospital or a physician specialist, there will be some amount of peer review of the initial primary care physician. Thus, although solo practice primary care physicians may appear to lack any formal connection with colleagues, they do not practice in a completely autonomous fashion as long as any patients are referred to colleagues.

It is possible, however, for poorly performing physicians to intentionally distribute their referrals to physician specialists, hospitals, and other health agencies so that no one professional or group of professionals has sufficient opportunity to recognize the consistent pattern of poor performance. That is, by careful selection of referrals the poorly performing solo family practitioners can minimize the risk of identification as such and subsequent informal or formal sanctions. Therefore, Freidson argues that the notion of "total autonomy" can realistically

Figure 1.2   Simplified decision-making and referral process for patients of primary care physicians

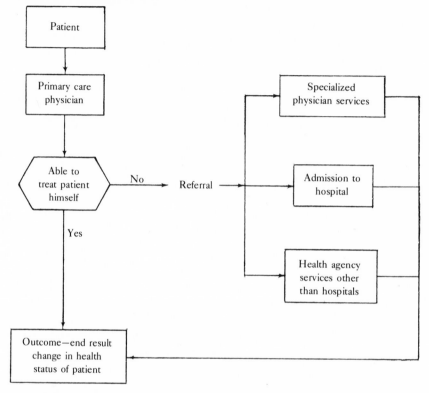

Source: S. M. Shortell, *A Model of Physician Referral Behavior: A Test of Exchange Theory in Practice.* Chicago: Center for Health Administration Studies, 1972. Reprinted with permission.

occur only under a limited set of circumstances which do not generally appear in American medicine. Thus, he perceives that physicians either band together, forming associations, partnerships, or groups, to minimize the "tyranny of client choice," or remain solo practitioners to minimize the "tyranny of colleague choice." Of course, minimizing the potential for one form of tyranny maximizes the potential for the other.

While the solo practice arrangement has been the tradition in the United States, with most physicians working in that type of practice setting through the 1960s, things began to change in the 1970s. Writing more than a decade and a half ago, Freidson (1970, 92) distinctly summarizes these changes:

> In the United States today, the supply of physicians in many areas is such that client control can be avoided; but increasingly, colleague control cannot. Dependence on

colleagues in one way or another is the rule today in the United States because consultations, hospitals, and capital equipment are essential to modern practice. In short, present practice is not solo: it embraces a large variety of organized relationships, most of which currently emphasize colleague rather than client controls.

Should physicians elect to band together to escape the tyranny of client choice, they have three general organizational options from which to choose: the association, the partnership, and the group practice.

An important question is how these cooperative (i.e., alternatives to solo practice) arrangements develop. Freidson (1970) and Hall (1946, 1949) have discussed how cooperative arrangements develop during the careers of physicians, and the interested reader is referred to their work. Such cooperative arrangements develop in part simply to add order to the continual entrance of new physicians into the system and the continual withdrawal of older physicians from the system. Cooperative arrangements, especially associations and partnerships, provide a mechanism for bringing order to these entrances and exits in a relatively predictable fashion that minimizes the threat of competition. Other factors that motivate the development of cooperative arrangements include the demand to obtain "coverage" when physicians want to take off an evening or a weekend, a vacation, or sick time.

In all these situations, some type of cooperative arrangement is necessary so that patients are not "lost," "stolen," or left unattended. As a result, colleague networks (described in detail by Hall 1946) initially develop for solo practitioners for the purpose of sharing coverage while minimizing the threat of stolen patients. Hall and Freidson suggest that, from the colleague networks in which physicians are involved, associations begin to emerge, which may subsequently develop into partnerships, which in turn may develop into group practices. Although several decades have passed since Hall and Freidson described the development of colleague networks and the informal development of professional careers, their work is, perhaps, even more appropriate for the 1980s when newly licensed physicians are entering a more competitive professional job market. Accordingly, the notion of "sponsorship" described by Hall and by Freidson is even more important in the development of physicians' careers today.

As indicated earlier, when physicians elect to band together with other physicians they have generally chosen from among three organizational options. The association has traditionally been the most common choice, because although it is a formal cooperative arrangement among physicians, colleagues are treated as peers and maintain their own patients separately. In the association, physicians share the expense of maintaining office facilities, equipment, and auxiliary personnel, while they maintain their own private patients. Practicing in closer proximity to colleagues and sharing auxiliary staff, however, facilitates more peer review than was possible in solo settings. Accordingly, the association represents the first step away from personal autonomy and toward peer review. The magnitude of that step, however, is not great, because only very limited economic factors are brought into play, and thus the enhanced access to informal information networks is not usually acted upon.

Quite similar in structure but not in effect is the small legal partnership, which usually comprises two physicians. They share not only the expenses of the office and auxiliary staff maintenance but profits as well. The particular method of dividing profits is almost always a matter of contention, especially among different medical specialties that may handle more or fewer patients with higher or lower fees. The most important distinction between the partnership and the association is that in the partnership each partner has a clear and definite monetary interest in the other partner. Accordingly, the increased flow of information and partner dependency makes the informal negative sanctions of the peer review process far more effective in the partnership.

The last type of practice setting is group practice, which is becoming more and more popular. In fact, about one physician in four actively practicing medicine is currently involved in group practice. This represents a considerable increase from the few thousand involved in group practice during the earlier part of the century (see figure 1.3). Although group practices have been rather extensively surveyed in recent years, there is no clear theoretical or empirical specification of the exact point at which the expanding partnership becomes a group practice. Indeed, Freidson (1970, 98) writes:

> the difference between a two- and a three-man partnership does not seem sociologically significant, nor does the difference between a two-man partnership and a three-man group. . . . If numbers are to be used to define group practice, . . . the minimum number of five full-time physicians seems reasonable. Five full-time physicians . . . can serve an ordinary population of anywhere from five to twenty thousand, depending on the proportion of general practitioners, internists, pediatricians, the financial arrangements with patients, and the general style of practice. As the number of patients and doctors increases further, it seems likely that, modified somewhat by the strength of the doctors' bargaining position, some of the technical characteristics of bureaucracy will emerge: hierarchical organization, extensive division of labor, systematic roles and procedures, and the like. In a logically ideal sense, this may be seen as a bureaucratic practice.

Thus, the distinction between a small partnership and a group practice may be seen more as a qualitative difference in the environment in which medicine is practiced than as a quantitative aspect of the number of physicians arbitrarily used to define a group practice. For example, the American Medical Association's definition of a group practice as three or more physicians seems somewhat arbitrary, given the difficulties involved in distinguishing a three-physician group from a three-physician partnership.

The important sociological and economic differences in the organization and function of medical practice are, among others, economies of scale, the likelihood

Figure 1.3   Number of physicians in group practice, 1932-1980

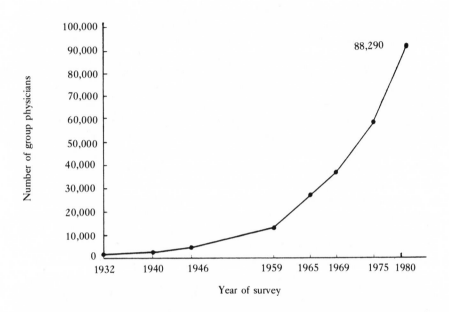

Adapted from: S. Henderson, R. Odem, and K. Ginsburg, *Medical Groups in the U.S., 1980.* Chicago: American Medical Association, 1982. Reprinted with permission.

for peer review, consultation, and the substitution of allied health services for physician services (Wolinsky 1982). Perhaps the most interesting of these is the differential probability for effective peer review of physicians, which may be considered synonymous with quality control as a generalized and self-imposed professional standards review organization (PSRO). In solo practice very little peer review occurs because physicians, by definition, work "autonomously" in isolation from their colleagues (especially in the case of the general practitioner). In group practice the situation is reversed: bureaucratic mechanisms make the information (case histories, medical charts, and complaints) necessary to institute and expedite peer review much more readily available. Moreover, the existence of malpractice liability and patient loss provide the fiscal incentive to control (i.e., review) poorly performing physicians in the profit-sharing group practice setting. Peer review in associations and partnerships essentially lies between that of solo and group practices; associations are closer to solo practice, and partnerships are closer to group practice.

Based on this decidedly organizational approach to human behavior (i.e., the preference for the nurture versus the nature explanation of human behavior), one can readily understand why the practice of medicine is expected to vary depending upon the practice setting. For example, in the client-dependent setting of solo practice (especially for the general practitioner) one would expect shorter patient queues and longer patient visits than in less client-dependent and more colleague-dependent settings. That is, for the more client-dependent settings, patient concerns and desires are more likely to be at center stage; in the colleague-dependent settings, the efforts to produce satisfaction are directed towards fellow professionals rather than actual consumers.

The bureaucratic nature of group practice may be expected to impose certain rules and regulations that constrain the physician's independence in the practice of medicine. For example, in group practice there may be more detailed protocols to be followed in a given situation than in solo practice, and in group practice there may be a more systematic method of keeping and annotating patient records. Moreover, in group practice there will more likely be a systematic method for the review of those records. Thus, it follows from Freidson's theory of the organization of medical practice that different practice settings will have different effects on patients and practitioners.

To the extent that patients and practitioners recognize that the practice of medicine will vary, depending on the setting in which it is delivered, both may seek out that practice setting which most closely reflects their preferences. For example, patients who prefer their physicians to be more responsive to their needs, whether those needs are medical or socio-emotional, may prefer to seek their medical care from solo practice physicians, because those solo practitioners will be more client-dependent. In contrast, patients who prefer more organized, systematic, and bureaucratic settings would be more likely to opt for group practices. Patients who wish to enjoy the benefits of both solo and group practice settings would probably choose the association or partnership settings.

Similarly, physicians whose most important preference is for personal autonomy would be most likely to favor solo practices in which they would be insulated from the scrutiny of their peers. Physicians whose most important preference is for medical responsibility would probably rather work in group practices in which peer review and professional concerns are likely to be maximized. As was the case for patients who preferred to strike a balance between the advantages of solo and group practice, physicians who desire a mixture of the medical responsibility of groups and the personal autonomy of solo practice are most likely to choose association or partnership settings.

When taken together, the preferences of patients and physicians for the advantages of certain practice settings suggest that there is likely to be some self-selection (for both patients and physicians) into medical practice settings. That is, in addition to the *nurture* effect of the practice setting on the practice of medicine, there is also likely to be a *nature* effect involving the self-selection of physicians who prefer solo practice into solo practice settings, of physicians who prefer group practice into group practice settings, and so forth. Thus, in assessing the effect of the organization of medical practice on the practice of medicine (i.e., nurture), the effects of self-selection (i.e., nature) must be statistically controlled. Otherwise, it would not be possible to determine whether a significant practice setting (i.e., nurture) effect has occurred.

The Correspondence of the Theory to Empirical Data

Although to date there have been no studies conducted that assess the full range of practice settings specified in Freidson's (1970) typology, there have been a number of reports comparing two or more practice settings with each other along some of the dimensions described above. Twenty-seven of these articles, all published since 1970, are of particular interest inasmuch as they provide some opportunity for limited evaluations of the typology's hypotheses. These articles have been grouped into five clusters based on their general orientation and correspondence to topics specifically addressed by Freidson, including:

1. general hypotheses and empirical evidence on solo versus group fee-for-service differences
2. comparisons of the practice of medicine from the physician's perspective across several practice settings
3. comparisons of the practice of medicine from the patient's perspective across several practice settings
4. the relationship between medical practice settings and client satisfaction
5. papers focusing on sociological influences on clinical decision making.

We shall briefly review the results of these 27 studies by cluster, focusing on the correspondence between their results and Freidson's typology.

Cluster One: Four Papers on Solo versus Group Practice

The first cluster of papers presents general hypotheses and evidence concerning solo versus group fee-for-service practice setting differences and contains four papers (Graham 1972; Mahoney 1973; Freshnock and Goodman 1979, 1980). Graham sets out to systematically identify whether or not the alleged potential benefits of group practice, which at that point had already appeared repeatedly in the literature, could be supported by existing evidence. In particular, Graham focuses on the issues of accessibility, quality, continuity, and efficiency. Although the available evidence usually supported group practice as a more advantageous form of medical care organization compared with solo practice on the dimensions of accessibility, quality, continuity, and efficiency, Graham (1972, 57–58) puts his remarks in perspective by stating:

> The supposed advantages of group practice collectively form an ideal construct. . . . Many of the advantages lack documented evidence; where evidence exists, certain advantages appear unrealized to the extent theoretically possible. These observations . . . suggest a number of possible intervening variables which can only be specified through such research, and bring to question the means for more fully realizing the potentials of group practice.

More importantly, Graham was one of the first to recognize that the alleged benefits of group practice might not accrue to all group practice settings. In effect, Graham argues that all group practice settings were not necessarily alike.

On another aspect of the difference between physicians in solo versus group fee-for-service practice, Mahoney (1973) was concerned mostly with how the characteristics of physicians differed between those settings. In particular, she hypothesized that the young physicians in her 1960–61 sample of 2,055 graduates of American medical schools would be influenced by three important factors in choosing a practice setting: general career plans, background attributes, and the nature of their medical education. Somewhat surprisingly, Mahoney found that neither the background attributes nor the nature of the young physicians' medical educations were significantly related to their plans for picking a practice setting. Moreover, Mahoney's (1973, 16) data suggest that young physicians view their initial practice setting choices basically as a "more or less irreversible decision, just as specialty choice is, rather than as a circumstance that might change as the nation's health needs change, or as the physician moves through different stages in his career." Thus, Mahoney concluded that the young physicians in her study viewed their first professional position as a career commitment to building a particular medical specialty *and* practice setting. The shortcoming of Mahoney's study is that the data are based on young physicians' plans for practice settings at the start and at the peak of their careers, rather than on actual observations of the types of practice settings in which this cohort of physicians began and ended their careers. Accordingly, it is not possible to determine how closely the young physicians' preferences (i.e., plans) matched the actual practice settings in which they started and subsequently developed their careers.

The two other studies in this cluster are those of Freshnock and Goodman (1979, 1980). In one study, Freshnock and Goodman (1980) developed a model of physician choice of practice setting which includes as predictors both the characteristics of individual physicians and the socioeconomic environment in which they practice. Their model of practice setting choice was then estimated separately for each of nine specialty groupings in order to control for and allow a comparison of interspecialty differences in practice setting choice. Using multivariate probit regression analysis on data from the American Medical Association's (AMA's) Masterfile of all physicians engaged in the practice of medicine, Freshnock and Goodman (1980, 28) were able to generate the following empirical profile of group practice physicians, regardless of their medical specialty:

> He is Board certified, a member of AMA, younger than 55 years of age, a graduate of a U.S. medical school, practices in a county with well-developed hospital services, a high hospital bed-to-population ratio, a high specialty-specific physician-to-population ratio, a low population density, and in a state with a relatively late year of entry into the United States.

Thus, Freshnock and Goodman were able to identify the pattern of significant differences between physicians in solo versus group practice settings. Perhaps most important was their identification of significant differences on *both* the physicians' own characteristics and the socioeconomic environment in which they practiced. Their results support the "developmental hypothesis," which suggests that independent of the characteristics of physicians, there are environmental constraints that may be more or less conducive to the formation of group versus solo practice settings.

In their other paper, Freshnock and Goodman (1979) examined why 25 percent of the group practices operating in the United States in 1969 had failed by 1975. Internal practice characteristics and external environmental variables were used as determinants of group practice survival, under the assumption that these variables are likely to influence the "adaptive capacity" of a group practice to satisfy its clients and thus affect the probability of the group's survival. Using data from the AMA's surveys of group medical practices in the United States in 1969 and 1975, Freshnock and Goodman (1979, 361) found that the internal factors were more likely to influence group survival than external environmental conditions, and that

> size is the most consistent determinant of group survival. However, corporate ownership, executive policy determination, number of secretaries employed, and group age evidence similar significant effects on survival.

Thus, their analysis was able to identify, at a general level, those factors that allowed group practices to be more adaptable to changing environmental conditions and as a result more likely to survive from 1969 to 1975. Because their study focused on the survival of group practices, however, they were not able to make inferences concerning differences in performance or the degree of survivability among the 75 percent of group practices that did survive. Nonetheless, Freshnock and Goodman were able to demonstrate that all group practices are not the same and that different configurations may have a considerable impact on the performance of those group practices.

Cluster Two: Ten Papers from the
Physician's Perspective

The second cluster of articles focuses on comparisons of medical practice across various practice settings from the physician's perspective (Mechanic 1975; Williamson 1975; Greenley and Kirk 1976; Perkoff 1978; Breslau, Novack, and Wolf 1978a, 1978b; Hull 1979; Luke and Thomson 1980a, 1980b; Roos 1980). Mechanic's (1975) study is by far the most comprehensive. It presents a fairly wide-ranging comparison of data on the practice of medicine between physicians in fee-for-service nongroup and group practices, as well as with physicians in prepaid group practices. The data are taken from two national surveys, the AMA's Periodic Survey of Physicians in 1970 and a comparable survey of physicians in group practice settings (using a sampling frame also provided by the AMA). Analysis of the data was limited to general practitioners and pediatricians, resulting in 113 general practitioners and 43 pediatricians in group fee-for-service practices, 606 general practitioners and 136 pediatricians in nongroup fee-for-service practice settings, and 108 general practitioners and 154 pediatricians in prepaid group practices.

Although he presents a variety of comparisons of sociodemographic and professional characteristics of the physicians, their workloads, and the environments in which they work, Mechanic's principal purpose was to compare and contrast the practice of medicine in prepaid versus nonprepaid settings. The theoretical model guiding Mechanic's (1975, 203) analysis may be best summarized as a "target-time" hypothesis, which suggests that

> doctors have a concept of how much time they ought to devote to their practice. For those paid on a salary or capitation basis, this concept is partially shaped by the fact that the doctor will have contractual obligations for a given number of sessions. Although doctors may adjust to varying patient demands in their practice, they do this within a range that they believe constitutes a reasonable and equitable work-week. If patient demand is large, the doctor must either practice in a more hurried way to get through the daily queue or increase the time he spends seeing patients.

Mechanic anticipated that physicians in prepaid practice settings would respond to increased patient demands by decreasing the amount of time that they spent per patient so that they would not have to increase their total patient care hours. Conversely, he anticipated that physicians in fee-for-service practice settings would hold constant the amount of time they spent per patient while increasing the total amount of time they spent seeing patients, thus expanding their work week.

The data support Mechanic's (1975, 203) hypothesis:

> Fee-for-service physicians spend more time in direct patient care activities than those in prepaid practice, and the best single predictor of income among fee-for-service physicians is the number of patients seen. In contrast, prepaid practices are likely to deal with increased patient demand by either delaying patient care, using the

queue as a rationing device, allowing the patient to see a specially available urgent care physician, or by scheduling patients with their physicians as extra patients. The additional load on the primary care physician who must see additional patients within his scheduled session results in a more assembly-line practice, one that hurries the doctor and makes him less responsive to the patient.

In part, this may explain the apparent anomaly that patients in prepaid practice settings generally report receiving the same or better quality care than they would have received in fee-for-service settings, although they concurrently report being less satisfied with the affective dimensions of that medical care. Mechanic argues that the different reimbursement incentives in prepaid practice settings result in a greater degree of indifference between patient and practitioner compared with the more traditional relationship found in fee-for-service settings. Thus, Mechanic's study is one of the first to point out that it is not merely the difference between solo versus group practice settings that results in differences in the practice of medicine; the practice of medicine also depends on the different methods of reimbursing physicians within group practice settings.

The nine remaining studies in this cluster generally follow a similar vein, although they treat much smaller ranges of medical practice differences. Williamson (1975) was concerned with the adoption of new pharmaceuticals among general practitioners in solo and group fee-for-service settings in England. His results indicate that physicians in group practice settings adopted new pharmaceuticals much more rapidly than their solo practice counterparts. Indeed, the difference between the average adoption time was about 25 weeks in favor of the group practice physicians. Moreover, when the average adoption time was calculated separately for solo physicians, three-physician groups, four-physician groups, and five- or six-physician groups, there was a very significant relationship such that the larger the group the faster the average adoption time. Although sample sizes were small and there were no physicians in "large" group practice settings, these data suggest that the maintenance of a high quality medical practice is easier in group as opposed to solo practice settings. That is, if the adoption of new, effective drugs can be considered an indicator of high quality medical practice, then Williamson's data demonstrate that it is easier to maintain high quality medicine in group practice than in solo practice.

Greenley and Kirk (1976) employed an exchange theory framework in reviewing a variety of studies on access to health care in different organizational settings. Their concern was that factors related to the organizational structure of practice settings might influence the identification of the personal and health problems to be treated, as well as the rates of those problems. Their review (1976, 321) suggests that "these treated incidence and prevalence rates are, in part, products of organizational factors rather than indicators of any true rates for a particular problem in the community." This finding has considerable importance for the analysis of the access issue, because it implies that utilization rates will in part depend on the mix of practice settings available to consumers. Thus, Greenley and Kirk provide additional evidence that the organization of medical practice influences the practice of medicine.

Similarly, Perkoff (1978) reviewed data from several different practice settings, all of which were responsible for providing care to prepaid enrollees. These data (1978, 638) led him to conclude that

> while much work needs to be done to define just which controlling factors in these organizations most directly affect the numbers of patients seen by different physicians, the data are consistent with the idea that the organization of medical care and the training of the physicians employed directly affect the pattern of medical care provided.

Thus, Perkoff was also able to demonstrate that the organization of medical practice affects the practice of medicine.

In two provocative papers, Breslau, Wolf, and Novack (1978a, 1978b) examined the relationship between physicians' task delegation and job satisfaction in traditional versus modern practice settings. The traditional practice setting included physicians in solo practices or in single specialty partnerships or small groups of two to five physicians. The modern practice settings were six large, complex medical care organizations that radically departed from the solo practice prototype. With regard to physicians' delegation of certain tasks to nonphysicians, Breslau, Wolf, and Novack (1978a, 381) found that "physicians in large, complex organizations on the average delegated more than physicians in small, independent practices." Thus, their data suggest that the amount and complexity of task delegation in bureaucratic settings will be greater than in more traditional settings. With regard to job satisfaction, Breslau, Novack, and Wolf's results (1978b, 860) strongly suggest that "physicians and paramedical workers in modern settings are less satisfied with their jobs than comparable groups in traditional practices." Thus, although task delegation may be more likely in modern (i.e., bureaucratic) practice settings, job satisfaction for both those who delegate tasks and those to whom the tasks are delegated is lower than in traditional practice settings. Accordingly, Breslau, Novack, and Wolf provide further evidence for the relationship between the organization of medical practice and the practice of medicine, as well as for the relationship between the organization of medical practice and physician satisfaction.

Hull (1979) used data on 93 physicians to identify personal characteristics, professional attitudes, training, and practice characteristics that were related to the use of psychiatric referrals by nonpsychiatric physicians. Hypothesizing that physicians in group practice settings would refer fewer psychiatric patients in each of a variety of diagnostic categories than would their counterparts in solo practice settings, Hull found that there was a significant difference only with regard to psychotic patients. The difference, however, was not as expected. That is, physicians in group practice settings were significantly more likely than their counterparts in solo practice settings to refer psychotic patients to psychiatrists. No additional significant differences were found between the referral patterns in solo and group practice settings.

Roos (1980) examined differences in the quality of care provided and in physicians' productivity between solo and group practice Canadian physicians. Her data (1980, 357) suggest that

> physicians in groups have different practice patterns than the solo practitioners, but the productivity and quality gains associated with group practice may be overstated. Practice patterns differ because group practitioners see larger numbers of different patients in a given year than do solo practitioners. This does not necessarily mean higher productivity.

Moreover, Roos failed to find any significant differences on a variety of quality of care measures between solo and group practice physicians. When taken together, the Hull and Roos studies suggest that while there may be some differences in the practice of medicine between solo and group practice settings, these differences may well be overstated, and that further research is necessary to resolve the issue.

In two papers, Luke and Thomson (1980a, 1980b) examined the differences between a prepaid and a fee-for-service group practice with regard to the use of within-hospital services and interphysician consulting patterns. Their study focused on the medical staff of a large, major short term general hospital in Denver, using data on 29 physicians in the prepaid and 21 physicians in the fee-for-service group practices. No significant differences were found between the two practice settings with regard to length of stay, laboratory charges, radiology charges, or total charges, although these utilization indicators were generally lower for the prepaid group. There were, however, significant differences between the two practice settings concerning the use of clinical resources. Luke and Thomson (1980a, 226) found that

> the prepaid group consistently engaged in the lowest level of consulting (both requesting and rendering) and fee-for-service group physicians engaged in the highest. . . . This indicates that the fee-for-service group structure reinforces the incentives facing physicians to generate and share in consultations, referrals and other forms of clinical services. . . . Prepaid group physicians were found to have the lowest request/render ratios for consulting *outside* of their group (i.e., with physicians in the fee-for-service group or with unaffiliated physicians) among the three categories of physicians.

Luke and Thomson (1980b) also report that the physicians in the prepaid group practice relied more on resident physicians as consultants and achieved a lower level of reciprocity in consulting exchange patterns than their counterparts in the fee-for-service group practice setting. Perhaps more interesting is the fact that physicians in both groups demonstrated a mutual avoidance of each other in selecting consulting partners. Although based on a small sample of physicians from just one hospital, the Luke and Thomson studies suggest that the structure of physicians' referral patterns is affected by the organization of medical practice and organizational norms apparently exist which differentially constrain the referral opportunities of physicians in prepaid versus fee-for-service group practice settings.

Cluster Three: Four Papers from the Patient's Perspective

The third cluster of articles shows comparisons of medical practice across several different practice settings from the patient's perspective (Shortell et al. 1977; Dutton 1979; Berkanovic, Telesky, and Reeder 1981; Burkett 1982). Shortell et al. assessed the interrelationships among patient characteristics, provider characteristics, and a variety of other measures related to the use of health services. Using data collected on 106 hypertension patients who were enrolled in the Seattle prepaid health care plan, Shortell et al. compared the 56 patients who received their care from a prepaid health plan with the 50 patients who received their care from a fee-for-service group practice. Using path analytic techniques, they found statistically significant differences between the practice settings on age-adjusted blood pressure levels, annualized visits to the doctor, continuity of care, and physician performance.

After identifying these additive effects on the use of health services, Shortell et al. then constructed separate regression models for the prepaid and fee-for-service patients. After finding that the characteristics of the individual patients were far more important in predicting utilization and satisfaction in the prepaid settings, they conclude that

> *the successful delivery of care in prepaid group practice settings depends greatly on the characteristics of the target group served,* such as family size, education, and sex, while in the independent fee-for-service system successful delivery of care tends to depend somewhat more on physician-related characteristics such as professional qualifications and specialty mix. (Shortell et al. 1977, 157)

Thus, they are able to demonstrate not only that the practice of medicine, from the patient's perspective, varies from practice setting to practice setting, but also that the importance of traditional predictors of health services utilization differ from one setting to another.

In a study of ambulatory care patterns in five different health care delivery systems in Washington, D.C., Dutton (1979) reaches similar conclusions. Comparing adjusted health services utilization levels in solo practice, fee-for-service group practice, prepaid group practice, public clinics, and hospital outpatient departments, Dutton (1979, 221) found that sources used primarily by the poor . . . contained important structural and financial barriers, and had the lowest rate of patient-initiated use. The prepaid system, in contrast, maximized patients' access to both preventive care and symptomatic care, and did not seem to inhibit physician-controlled follow-up care. The results suggest some perverse effects of fee-for-service payment: patients, especially poor patients, appear to be deterred from seeking preventive and symptomatic care, while physicians were encouraged to expand follow-up services.

Thus, Dutton is also able to demonstrate significant differences in the use of health services based on the health care delivery system to which the patient had access. Moreover, Dutton (1979, 239) views these data as a reflection of the inequitable nature of the present health care delivery system:

> The more desirable systems will be used by the more privileged members of society, while the less desirable systems are allocated to the less privileged. . . . A pluralistic health care system may provide varied options for the affluent, but in the light of present social realities, it is unlikely to do so for the poor.

In essence, Dutton warns that although prepaid group practice may provide more comprehensive and higher quality health care, it is more likely to be made available to the affluent. The likely result will be to increase the gap between the quality of care received by the affluent and that received by the less fortunate.

Using data from the Los Angeles Health Survey, Berkanovic, Telesky, and Reeder (1981) focused on structural and psychosocial factors related to the decision to seek medical care for specific symptoms. They used a hierarchical multiple regression design to isolate the net effects of five sets of variables, including need, social structure, the organization of care, general social network patterns and health orientation, and social network influences and personal beliefs about the symptoms. Although their regression model was able to explain 57 percent of the variance in the decision to seek medical care, the need factors, network influences, and personal beliefs about the symptoms accounted for 54 percent of the total variance. Thus, the sets of social structure and organization of care variables accounted for only 3 percent of the variance in the decision to seek medical care. Accordingly, Berkanovic, Telesky, and Reeder's results fail to support the hypothesis that the organization of medical practice has an impact on a patient's decision to seek medical care for symptoms. Their findings may, however, be due to the crudity with which the structure and organization factors were measured.

Using data obtained from one independent practice association (IPA) model HMO that involved 130 primary care physicians in 62 medical offices (as well as an extensive panel of specialists), Burkett (1982) examined variations in physician utilization patterns between the IPA offices. Hypothesizing that practice patterns in IPA offices which had a larger number of HMO patients and a longer history of participation in the IPA would conform most closely with the traditional HMO cost control objectives, Burkett reported some startling findings.

Although health services utilization was found to be related to medical specialty, it was not related either to the HMO patient load or to the length of membership in the IPA. Indeed, a significant positive relationship was found between the age of the IPA office and hospitalization rates, such that the longer the physician's office had been part of the IPA the higher the hospital utilization rate. A similar relationship was found for the use of referral services. Burkett suggests, however, that these data may actually reflect a self-selection problem that arose in the recent past, when changes in the recruitment and admission of physicians into this particular IPA occurred.

Cluster Four: Five Papers on
Client Satisfaction

The fourth cluster of studies assesses the effect of medical practice settings on a variety of dimensions of client satisfaction (Tessler and Mechanic 1976; Gray 1980; Ross, Wheaton, and Duff 1981; Ross and Duff 1982; Ross, Mirowsky, and Duff 1982). Tessler and Mechanic (1976) present a comprehensive comparison of consumer satisfaction between 354 individuals who used Blue Cross (fee-for-service) practice settings and 356 persons who received their health care from prepaid group practices. Although the vast majority of respondents in both practice settings were very satisfied with the medical care they and their families received, there were significantly lower levels of consumer satisfaction with care in the prepaid practice settings. Satisfaction levels were also found to be related to marital status, skepticism toward medical care, psychological well-being, and perceived health status. When these additional correlates of consumer satisfaction were statistically controlled, significant differences between the practice settings remained, with those in the prepaid settings reporting a greater degree of dissatisfaction.

Another interesting finding emerged when Tessler and Mechanic questioned the respondents about their perceptions of accessibility to health care. The prepaid enrollees reported longer patient queues associated with appointment scheduling, but shorter patient queues upon arrival at the physician's office, than their fee-for-service counterparts. Tessler and Mechanic (1976, 112–13) argue:

> These results suggest a kind of tradeoff between the scheduling of appointments and waiting time upon arrival. The prepaid plan may have adhered to a rigid appointment schedule, while fee-for-service physicians may have been more willing to try to squeeze people in even at the price of long waiting periods in the doctor's office. The two delivery systems appear to be dealing with a common problem (too many consumers relative to the supply of health care personnel) in different ways, with prepaid practice eliciting more consumer complaints in relation to scheduling appointments and fee-for-service physicians eliciting more consumer complaints in relation to waiting time upon arrival.

Thus, although Tessler and Mechanic conclude that there were statistically significant differences in consumer satisfaction between the two practice settings, the strengths and liabilities of each may be equally offsetting. That is, in both practice settings patient queues were used at one and the same time to ration access to health care as well as to satisfy consumers.

In a similar study, Gray (1980) used data from the Federal Employee's Health Benefits Program Utilization Study. She compared consumer satisfaction with physician services among 390 enrollees in a prepaid group practice with that among 421 enrollees in a Blue Cross/Blue Shield system. Significantly more of the fee-for-service patients were completely satisfied with the doctor's quality of care, courtesy, follow-up care, and personal interest in them, than were their prepaid group practice counterparts. Moreover, although the differences between the two practice settings were not significant with regard to the amount of time the doctor spent with the patient, how much information the doctor provided to the patient, or the doctor's explanation of home care, a larger percentage of the fee-for-service patients were, again, more satisfied than their prepaid group practice counterparts. Thus, Gray's results replicate Tessler and Mechanic's (1976) on two issues: the generally high level of consumer satisfaction regardless of practice setting, and the higher satisfaction levels among fee-for-service patients. Gray suggests that these differences in consumer satisfaction might be diminished if physicians in prepaid practice settings would modify their patient management approaches and become more personal or affable.

In a provocative set of papers, Ross and her colleagues (Ross, Wheaton, and Duff 1981; Ross and Duff 1982; Ross, Mirowsky, and Duff 1982) examine the relationship between consumer satisfaction and client characteristics, organizational characteristics, and characteristics of the doctor-client interaction. Of particular interest to our study are their findings on the effects of the organization of medical practice. Analyzing data based on 372 cases for which information was available on the mother, her child, the pediatrician involved, and an observed visit of the child with the pediatrician, Ross and her colleagues (Ross, Wheaton, and Duff 1981, 243) set out to test a theoretical model in which

> *expectations* about medical care and *experiences* with care counteract each other. Specifically, clients enter HMOs and other large prepaid groups with negative expectations, whereas they enter solo practice with positive expectations. However, their experiences with the medical care in solo practice tend to be negative compared with the experiences of clients in large groups.

The data (Ross, Wheaton, and Duff 1981, 252) support their hypothesis, leading them to state

> In large prepaid groups, clients have images of the impersonal "clinic" doctor, a doctor who treats the poor, and who is uncaring and rushed. These images are generally held and they produce negative expectations about the care received in "clinics."

These expectations produce relative dissatisfaction in clients who have recently joined a large prepaid group. However, as positive experiences in these groups accumulate, satisfaction increases. The picture is reversed for the clients of solo practitioners.

Speculating about relationships in both partnerships and small groups, they suspect that clients enter these settings with average satisfaction levels and thus are not terribly surprised with the care that they receive.

Collapsing their practice setting variables into a simple dichotomy, Ross and her colleagues assessed the impact of practice settings on the number of visits to the physician, as well as on the relationship of physician status characteristics to client satisfaction. They report (Ross and Duff 1982) a significant practice setting effect on pediatrician utilization. Children in prepaid group practice settings averaged slightly more than one visit per year more than children in solo fee-for-service, small group, or partnership settings, even after statistically adjusting for a variety of socioeconomic and health status characteristics. With regard to effect of practice settings on the relationship between physician status characteristics and client satisfaction, Ross, Mirowsky, and Duff (1982, 317) hypothesize that

in small fee-for-service practices such as solo practices, where the client chooses his or her physician, status characteristics of the doctor would be unrelated to client satisfaction. Conversely, in large prepaid group practices where the client is assigned a physician, nonnormative physician status characteristics would create lower client satisfaction.

The data support this hypothesis as well.

When taken together, the studies of Ross and her colleagues

1. replicate previous studies reporting higher levels of client satisfaction in fee-for-service settings compared with prepaid group practice settings

2. demonstrate more ambulatory care utilization in prepaid practices than in fee-for-service settings

3. suggest that while having a non-WASP (White Anglo-Saxon Protestant) or non-Jewish physician in a prepaid group practice decreases client satisfaction levels, it does not do so in solo practice settings.

The latter provides some support for the self-selection of patients into practice settings. In the solo practice setting, likes (patients and physicians with the same religious status) attract each other; in the prepaid practice setting, patients may arbitrarily be assigned a physician whose religious status conflicts with theirs (i.e., whose religious status is nonnormative).

Cluster Five: Four Papers on
Sociological Influences

The last cluster of papers focuses on sociological influences on clinical decision making. In the first paper, Eisenberg et al. (1974) considered the intriguing question of whether or not the same physicians would practice medicine the same way in a prepaid and a fee-for-service practice setting. To address this question, they collected data from the practices of four pediatricians who were associated with the Medical Care Group of Washington University and who were also associated with a fee-for-service pediatric group practice. During an eight-week period, 277 pediatric patient encounters were observed in the prepaid setting, and the same number of encounters per pediatrician were studied in the fee-for-service setting. Thus, it was possible to examine whether or not the same pediatricians practiced medicine differently in the prepaid setting and in the fee-for-service setting. The data indicate that significantly more laboratory studies were ordered in the prepaid practice setting, all four pediatricians referred a significantly greater number of their prepaid patients to other specialists, and a significantly greater number of prepaid practice patients received allergy injections.

Further analyses suggest that about half of the differences in laboratory procedures could be accounted for by the presence of laboratory equipment on site in the prepaid practice, and that the difference in allergy injections was probably related to having a nurse practitioner available in the prepaid setting. However, even after taking these issues into consideration, there were still significant differences in the number of laboratory procedures ordered and in the number of consultations requested. The most likely interpretation is that the differences accrued as a result of two factors: differences in the organizational setting and the lack of financial barriers in the prepaid practice (which did not place patients at risk for the additional lab tests that were ordered).

In a subsequent paper, Eisenberg (1979) reviews the increasing scrutiny that clinical decision making has undergone in recent years. Most of that scrutiny has concerned normative and quantitative dimensions of patterns in clinical decision making. Eisenberg (1979, 957) explores sociological influences on the decision-making process and identifies four specific sets of factors which influence the clinician's judgment:

> . . . the characteristics of the patient; the characteristics of the clinician; the clinician's interaction with his profession and the health care system; and the clinician's relationship with the patient.

The physician's interaction with his profession is the most interesting for this study. Citing Freidson's (1970) distinction between client- and colleague-dependent practices, Eisenberg concisely reviews the available literature on the effect of the organization of medical practice on clinical decision making. That literature, however, is very sparse. Moreover, Eisenberg (1979, 962) cites a number of flaws in the existing literature, including:

1. Few studies have been methodologically sound.

2. Seldom have there been controls for case mix or the severity of disease.

3. Often there have been no statistical analyses of the data.

4. Frequently the reports are more polemical than scholarly.

5. Multivariate analyses are seldom employed to control for confounding variables.

6. Most of the studies deal with psychiatric decision making, leaving considerable doubt about their generalizability to more typical medical decision-making situations.

Two studies by Rhee and his colleagues (Rhee 1977; Rhee, Luke, and Culverwell 1980) appear to have avoided most of the shortcomings identified by Eisenberg (1979). Using data from 454 physicians and their patients in 22 short-term general hospitals in Hawaii, Rhee (1977) sought to directly compare the effects of internal characteristics (nature effects, or the socialization and personality issues) with those of external characteristics (nurture effects, or the organizational setting). Using multiple correlation analyses, Rhee examined the net contributions of the internal and external characteristics toward explaining physician performance, which was operationalized as compliance with medical norms for the provision of care in offices and hospitals. The direct effects of the internal characteristics accounted for only 2 percent of the variance in the quality of physician performance, while the direct effects of the external characteristics accounted for nearly 10 percent. This provides considerable support for Freidson's lament that the nature argument has been overemphasized at the same time that the nurture argument has been underplayed. Rhee (1977, 10) concluded that

> physicians' present working environments had more influence on the quality of care than did their formal medical training, which implies that variation in present behaviors is more an outcome of the characteristics of the work situation than of what people have earlier internalized.

In the second paper, Rhee, Luke and Culverwell (1980) examined 3,316 hospital episodes taken from the same 22 general hospitals. The focus here was on determining whether a relationship existed between the degree of client versus colleague dependency in the practice setting and the medical care received by their patients. The data (Rhee, Luke and Culverwell 1980, 829) indicate that patients treated by more colleague-dependent (i.e., specialized) physicians received

> 1) higher scores on an index of quality of care; 2) more justified admissions; 3) more appropriate lengths of stay; 4) fewer overstays; but 5) more understays.

These findings provide further support for the effect that the informal structures of physicians' practices have on the way that they practice medicine. Moreover, these data suggest that the more colleague dependent the practice setting, the more likely there will be self-imposed peer review. Thus, the odds for the provision of higher quality medical care are enhanced in colleague-dependent practices.

The Evidence on Self-Selection

The literature reviewed above demonstrates that the practice of medicine does depend upon the organization of medical practice, although not always exactly as Freidson's (1970) typology would suggest. None of the studies cited, however, seriously considered or statistically controlled for the possibility of self-selection by the physician. (For an excellent review of the self-selection issue from the patient's perspective, see Berki and Ashcraft 1980.) Thus, while these studies have broadly shown the importance of the nurture argument by demonstrating observed differences between the practice of medicine in various practice settings, they have assumed that the self-selection of physicians into the different practice settings has not been an important factor in the practice of medicine in those settings. This is not surprising, as there are only four studies that have addressed the potential self-selection issue of physicians into different practice settings (McElrath 1961; Mechanic 1975; Mick et al. 1983; Wolinsky 1982). Moreover, in three of these the self-selection issue has, at best, been addressed tangentially or limited by the very nature of the study itself. In order to explore the potential implications of the self-selection issue, we shall review these four studies, concentrating on the most comprehensive one.

In the first study, McElrath (1961) examined the attitudes of 46 physicians in a prepaid group practice, dividing them into two groups based on the percentage of their patients for whom reimbursement was prepaid. His focus was on demonstrating that physicians with high levels of participation in prepaid group practice would have a different orientation than physicians with low levels. McElrath found that the physicians with higher levels of participation in the prepaid group practice favored pooling practice incomes and being in a group practice organization. In addition, the physicians who were heavily engaged in prepaid practice felt that their patients overused their services.

In a similar yet more detailed study, Mechanic (1975) compared general practitioners and pediatricians in prepaid group practices with their counterparts in fee-for-service group practices and in nongroup fee-for-service settings. Mechanic examined the differences between the physicians in the three practice settings in terms of their attitudes towards health and social policy issues. He found that the prepaid group practice physicians were more favorably disposed to the federal financing of health care and to the salaried reimbursement of physicians. Perhaps most interesting was the finding that the prepaid group practice physicians were more willing to recognize the problem of medical responsibility (i.e., the difficulty of uncertainty in medical decision making). Unfortunately, Mechanic's results are presented merely as an aside in his demonstration of the differences in the practice of medicine in prepaid group practice settings versus fee-for-service group practice settings.

The third study (Mick et al. 1983) actually compared physicians who elected to remain in prepaid group practices with those who left. Mick et al. found that those who left the prepaid group practice were more likely to believe that it inhibited their autonomy, their independence, and their professional development. Thus, they demonstrated that those who leave prepaid group practice have different attitudes from those who remain. They were not able, however, to address the issue of why physicians joined the prepaid group practice in the first place.

This leads us to the fourth study, which is the only one to date that has directly addressed the issue of why physicians choose different practice settings. Building upon an extension of Freidson's theory of the organization of medical practice described above, Wolinsky (1982) set out to assess what effect physicians' preferences for personal autonomy and medical responsibility had on their selection of a practice setting, apart from the effects of other characteristics known to be related to the choice of a practice setting. In his analysis of data on 4,500 physicians in different practice settings, Wolinsky defined medical practice selection as a function of the sociodemographic characteristics of the physicians, the characteristics of the environment in which they practiced, and their attitudes. The sociodemographic characteristics of the physician included age, sex, membership in the AMA, specialty board certification, and medical specialty; these characteristics were thought to predispose the physician to select either solo or group practice settings. The environmental characteristics, which were assumed to constrain a physician's opportunity to choose between the various practice settings, included the hospital bed ratio, location in a metropolitan area, average household income, and geographic location. Attitudes were measured by asking the physicians to indicate how important personal autonomy, professional contacts, earnings potential, the predictability of scheduling, the business side of practice, the quality of patient care, personal associations or friendships, and practice location were in choosing a practice setting. (For two similar treatments of this issue using the same data, see Goodman and Swartwout 1984 and Goodman and Wolinsky 1982.)

The results from multiple regression analyses indicate that the sociodemographic, environmental (except in the case of small group practice choices), and attitudinal characteristics do have significant impacts on the selection of medical practice settings. The sociodemographic characteristics indicate that physicians choosing solo practice are more likely to be older, not board certified, and not AMA members, while those opting for large group practices are more likely to be younger and board certified. Physicians selecting small group practices are more likely to be younger, male, board certified, and AMA members.

The impact of the vector of medical specialties indicates that physicians in general practice, internal medicine, surgery, obstetrics and gynecology, and psychiatry are more likely to choose solo practices. Pediatricians and radiologists are more likely to favor the small group setting, with radiologists also practicing in large groups. General practitioners, surgeons, obstetricians and gynecologists, and psychiatrists appear to avoid large group practices. These results reflect the affinity of the various medical specialties for the different medical practices. That is, psychiatrists opt for solo practice (because the nature of their work does not readily lend itself to patient sharing), radiologists tend toward small or large group practices (typically in hospitals which underwrite the expense of laboratory equipment through formal and informal arrangements), pediatricians choose small group settings (to share weekend and late-night calls), and the remaining primary care and surgical specialists have solo practices.

Among the environmental characteristics, the results indicate that solo practices are more common in underserved areas (those with lower hospital bed to population ratios) and are less common in the western United States where large group practices (especially HMOs) are the most developed. The reverse is true with respect to large group practices.

The effect of the attitudinal characteristics clearly supports the self-selection issue. That is, as expected, these data indicate that the attitudinal structure of physicians choosing solo medical practice is oriented principally toward the importance of personal autonomy. To a lesser extent, it is also focused on the *un*importance of the quality of medical care, professional and personal interactions, and the business side of medical practice. Thus, physicians who choose solo practice appear to be very concerned with personal autonomy, perhaps to the point that they consider the quality of care and other professional concerns unimportant in making the medical practice setting choice or believe that these issues do not vary by practice setting and are thus unimportant.

At the same time, and as expected, the results indicate that physicians opting for large group practices consider the quality of medical care, professional contacts, and the business side of medical practice important in choosing a medical practice. For them, personal friendships, personal autonomy, and earnings potential are unimportant in the decision-making process. Thus, physicians entering large group practices appear to be motivated by more professional and less personal factors.

Also as expected, physicians who choose small group practices appear to be between their solo and large group practice counterparts on the importance of these issues. Small group physicians consider the quality of patient care, personal friendships, and predictability in scheduling important factors in their decisions. For them, personal autonomy is unimportant. When coupled with the effects of medical specialty, this indicates that physicians opting for small group practices would prefer personal or friendly partnerships and associations which they believe permit them to provide better quality care while increasing the schedulability of their practices.

Wolinsky draws two conclusions from these data. First, in examining the selection of a medical practice one cannot simply contrast solo with group practice choices. Rather, one must examine the full range of practice settings either in terms of the four types originally described by Freidson or the three types in the refinement of that scheme that he suggested. There are important theoretical and empirical differences between small groups and large groups in addition to those between solo practice and group practice. These differences are lost when one assumes all groups to be equal, much as the differences between HMOs are lost when they are assumed to be equal.

Second, Wolinsky concludes that the sociodemographic, environmental, and attitudinal characteristics of physicians have significant impacts on their selection of medical practices. Although his data are clearly not definitive, it appears that the attitudinal characteristics, especially the importance of personal autonomy, are the most important in choosing a medical practice. That is, the hierarchical addition of the attitudinal characteristics into the equation approximately doubles the explained variance obtained when just the sociodemographic and environmental characteristics are used, regardless of whether the practice setting choice involves the solo setting, the small group setting, or the large group setting.

Wolinsky's (1982) study demonstrates one of the major problems of comparing the practice of medicine across various medical practice settings. In particular, his findings suggest that physicians who are more concerned with the quality of care and other professional issues select large group practice settings. That is, Wolinsky's findings question whether it is the HMO which leads to less personal patient-practitioner relationships and better quality medical care or whether these detriments and benefits result from physician's self-selection (or perhaps adverse selection) into HMOs versus solo or small group practices. Similarly, the reverse may be true in the solo practice setting, while those self-selecting into small group practices strike a balance between these extremes. Accordingly, future studies of the effect of the organization of medical practice on the practice of medicine should control for physician preferences (as a proxy for self-selection). Without such controls, it is not possible to assess accurately the advantages of one medical practice setting over another.

The importance of Wolinsky's (1982) study, however, must be tempered by three acknowledged design shortcomings. First, his data do not provide detailed information on either the small or large groups themselves. Thus, the particular structural configurations that exist among the medical groups are not known. Therefore, his model does not take into account the structural characteristics that may affect the physicians' selection of a particular type of medical practice.

Second, the items that Wolinsky used to tap the attitudinal characteristics may contain sufficient measurement error to make them somewhat difficult to interpret. The attitudinal measures simply asked physicians to rate several issues in their decision to go into solo versus group practice as very important, important, or not important. Thus, while we know how important these issues are to the choice of a practice setting, we do not know whether the physicians' practice settings actually maximized their preferences. For example, although physicians may report that personal autonomy is very important in their selection of a solo versus group practice setting, it does not necessarily follow that the practice which they selected maximized their personal autonomy.

Finally, the physicians that Wolinsky studied were, on average, 50 years old. Many of them were indicating reasons for practice setting choices that they had made several years earlier. Thus, it is impossible to determine whether the patterns found in those data resulted from changes in attitude in response to their socialization experiences in the practice settings (i.e., were they socialized into this attitudinal configuration?), or whether they were retrospectively justifying the choices that they had made (i.e., were they minimizing cognitive dissonance?). Despite these limitations, however, Wolinsky's study does demonstrate the importance of the self-selection of physicians into medical practice settings when the purpose of the research is to assess differences in the practice of medicine across practice settings. That is, his work suggests that in testing the effects of the *nurture* factors specified in Freidson's theory of the organization of medical practice, the *nature* factors associated with the self-selection of physicians into those practice settings must be statistically controlled whenever possible.

The Emergence of HMOs and Their Effect on the Practice of Medicine

Although some prepaid medical practices existed at the time that Freidson (1970) first presented his typology, that type of practice setting was rather uncommon. It was only mentioned in passing in the original typology (see Freidson 1970, 101–105). Since 1970, however, the growth and importance of prepaid practices has increased significantly. Indeed, in 1971 a new term for prepaid practice — "health maintenance organization" (HMO) — was introduced (Ellwood 1971), and HMOs were made an official national policy goal (Nixon 1971). The recognition and favored position of HMOs was formalized at the federal level in 1973 with the passage of the HMO Act (PL 93–222), solidified in 1974 by the National Health Planning and Resources Development Act (PL 93–641), and elaborated further by several subsequent amendments (Department of Health, Education, and Welfare 1974, 1975; PL 94–460; PL 95–559). Accordingly, one would assume that by now we would have a common understanding of what HMOs are, how they are supposed to affect the practice of medicine, and what and how well they actually do affect the practice of medicine. This, however, is not the case, as the literature reviewed above indicates.

The literature on the promise and performance of HMOs is somewhat paradoxical. On the one hand, it is quite extensive. On the other hand, it is not at all definitive. This dilemma is reflected by the fact that several informative but not necessarily consistent reviews of this voluminous literature already exist. It would seem, therefore, most appropriate to highlight the findings and conclusions reached in these extant reviews briefly, rather than present yet another review of the HMO literature itself. In doing so we shall focus on the evidence for whether or not HMOs affect the practice of medicine, and if so, how this occurs. Such an approach should set the stage for incorporating this new practice setting into Freidson's typology.

In an early review, Klarman (1963) used data collected between 1950 and 1961 to assess the effects of prepaid group practice on hospital use. (The term HMO had not yet been coined.) A simple comparison of hospitalization days per 1,000 members per year showed that during 1950 the rate of use in prepaid plans ranged between 490 and 685 days, while in Blue Cross plans the rate was 888 days, and for the United States population as a whole the rate was 1,165 days. By the year 1960–61 the rates in prepaid group practice plans had risen somewhat, ranging from 544 to 730 days, with Blue Cross rates rising markedly to 1,060 days, and the rate for the United States population rising to 1,265 days. Klarman considered nine theoretical explanations for the differences between hospitalization rates in prepaid group practice and in conventional health insurance plans. The explanations included differences in (1) the range of benefits, (2) the availability of ambulatory care services, (3) access to hospital beds, (4) the possibility of skimping on medical care in the prepaid plans by failing either to diagnose or to treat existing medical conditions, (5) physician reimbursement, (6) physician control over hospitalization, (7) the role and use of specialists, (8) the willingness of primary care physicians to provide private home health care, and (9) the length of patient stays. After considering these explanations in turn, Klarman (1963, 963–64) concludes:

> Of increasing prominence today is the presence or absence of controls. Controls take various forms and may be carried out by salaried physicians, by subscribers confronted with financial deterrents, or by self-insured plans in which the members actively cooperate; or controls may, in effect, be imposed by lack or inaccessibility of hospital beds. The organizational framework of group practice may constitute a source of control over hospital use, as well as a vehicle for providing ambulatory services.

In essence, Klarman attributes the effect to the differences in the controls that influence the organization, the physician, and the patient.

Reviewing basically the same data as Klarman, Weinerman (1964, 880) focuses on patients' perceptions of group medical care, arguing that "the proof of group practice must lie, after all, in the satisfaction of those who use its special type of service." He found that those enrolled in prepaid group practice were significantly more likely to express complaints concerning "waiting times, inadequate explanations by doctors, difficulty in getting house calls, and lack of interest in the patient as a person" (Weinerman 1964, 885). From these data he distilled the nature of the patient perception problem and cast it in sociological terms (Weinerman 1964, 886):

> The local practitioner is pictured as more ready to accommodate the patients' wants . . . whereas the structure of group practice is seen as bending the previously conditioned member to its doctor-oriented rules of procedure.

Weinerman (1964, 887–88) goes on to sketch the implications of the problem:

> Most importantly, the attitudes of patients—whether rational or not—profoundly affect the degree to which the program succeeds in its function, that of protecting its members' health. . . . The uneaten specialty on the dinner plate in the most excellent of restaurants makes little contribution either to nutrition or appetite.

In essence, Weinerman offers a radically different explanation for the smaller number of hospitalization days in prepaid group practice. He implies that it might not be the greater efficiency in prepaid group practice; rather, that such alternative health care delivery systems were just so much less "acceptable" (in terms of the expected and traditionally personal patient-practitioner relationship) that they resulted in a decline in health services utilization.

Donabedian's (1969) review is more comprehensive than either Klarman's or Weinerman's, and was prepared without reference to them in order to maintain an independent view. Donabedian studied choice of plan, subscriber satisfaction, utilization of ambulatory and hospital services, and the quality of care. He concludes that the major reasons that individuals enroll in a prepaid group practice plan (when given the choice through employee benefits) are geographic proximity, not having a private physician as a regular source of care, not being ideologically opposed to "socialized medicine," and the wider range of benefits. Once the employees had chosen membership in prepaid group plans, they were likely to complain about the impersonality of care, the clinic or charity medical care atmosphere, long waiting periods to see a physician, and the difficulty of obtaining house calls. In contrast, the same subscribers felt that they received good quality medical care in the prepaid group practice, but credited the quality to the availability of technical, diagnostic, and consultative resources rather than to the quality of the physicians themselves. With regard to utilization, Donabedian (1969, 11) argues that "the key question is not what is the level of utilization that is associated with any system of organizing care but what precisely happens to utilization and why." In other words, the utilization question should ask whether the utilization rate is appropriate rather than what the actual rate is. After an analysis stratified according to disease category (even though the data did not provide a clear answer to the question), Donabedian (1969, 15) concludes that

> the findings are consistent with the conclusion that (conventional insurance plans) over-hospitalize for the common respiratory conditions and the more minor surgical conditions such as benign neoplasms, tonsillectomies and accidental injuries.

In addition to showing that the prepaid plans reduced costs (through lowered hospitalization rates) while maintaining appropriate levels of utilization, the data indicated further cost reductions from the substitution of cheaper ancillary services for the more expensive physician services (also where appropriate). Overall, Donabedian (1969, 24–25) presents a very strong case for

> the capability of prepaid group practices to achieve a more rational pattern in the use of medical resources, its ability to control costs, and the greater protection it generally offers against the unpredictable financial ravages of illness.

Building on the earlier reviews, and making ample use of the massive data resources of the Kaiser Foundation Hospitals' Health Services Research Center, Greenlick (1972) assessed the impact of prepaid group practice on American medicine. As in the previous studies, he concluded that comprehensive coverage at a reasonable premium was the major attraction bringing subscribers into prepaid group practices. Greenlick (1972, 110) also found that

> the expenditures for providing medical care services for a total population covered by prepaid group practice programs are less than the expenditures for care to similar populations covered in the traditional individual fee-for-service system.

The reduced cost, however, could not be attributed to efficiencies of scale, but rather arose from "system efficiencies," such that

> by integrating the financing and the organization of medical care, PGP can reduce incentives for the physician or the population to prefer that equivalent services be provided on an in-patient rather than on an out-patient basis. (Greenlick 1972, 110)

In essence Greenlick concluded that, although all the data were not yet in, it was clear that prepaid group practices had several major advantages over conventional plans, the advantages stemming from the different incentives placed before physicians and patients alike.

Building on Donabedian's, Klarman's, and Weinerman's reviews, and updating them with data from more recent studies, Roemer and Shonick (1973) prepared an extensive review of HMO performance. They focused their review on subscriber composition, participation of physicians, utilization rates, quality assessments, costs and productivity, health status outcomes, and patient attitudes. After reviewing the data, Roemer and Shonick (1973, 271) conclude

> The "prepaid group practice" (PGP) model of HMO continues to yield lower hospital use, relatively more ambulatory and preventive service, and lower overall costs (counting both premiums and out-of-pocket expenditures) than conventional open-market fee-for-service systems. Economies of scale are still not proved. New data point to reduced disability from the PGP model of HMO, as well as to more favorable consumer attitudes (based mainly on the economic advantage, in spite of certain impersonalities of clinics) than exist toward conventionally insured private solo practice. The medical care foundation (individual practice association) . . . has yielded some evidence of economies of physician's care, but none in hospital use.

Having built up HMOs as the answer to the crisis in health care, Roemer and Schonick then go on to identify the two "principal hazards" that are inherent to the HMO concept: (1) the notion of inequitable "risk" selection, in which the HMO accepts as enrollees only the healthy, for whom the provision of health care is relatively inexpensive; and (2) the provision of poorer quality care through skimping. Moreover, these authors warn that once HMOs move into the mainstream of American health care it will become even more important to maintain vigilance to detect these two hazards, because both the critical approach to a new idea and the self-regulation of a new industry will wear off.

Gaus, Cooper, and Hirschman (1976) examined enrollment selectivity, utilization of services, accessibility of care, and patient satisfaction in ten HMOs serving Medicaid patients as opposed to the fee-for-service Medicaid population. With respect to utilization, they found a significant difference in hospitalization only for staff and group models, not for individual practice associations (IPAs). They concluded

> that capitation payment to an HMO alone is not significant enough to produce major changes in utilization and that organized multi-specialty group-practice arrangements with largely salaried physicians may be more significant. (Gaus, Cooper, and Hirschman 1976, 3)

This indicates that some incentives (those related to the organizational delivery of care) are more effective than others (those related to financing). Gaus, Cooper, and Hirschman also found that original health status, the use of ambulatory services (including preventive services), patient satisfaction, and access were remarkably similar in both the general Medicaid population and the HMOs.

In several recent papers, Luft (1978a, 1978b, 1979, 1980, 1981) has presented the most detailed and critical reviews of the literature on HMO performance to date. In particular, from a comprehensive review of the primary literature he has focused on the performance issues of how HMOs actually save money, why they appear to provide more preventive services, and whether they actually lower the rate of growth of medical care costs. Demonstrating that total costs (both premiums and out-of-pocket expenditures) are from 10 to 40 percent lower in HMOs than in conventional health insurance plans, Luft (1978a, 1336) notes that

> Most of the cost differences are attributable to hospitalization rates about 30 percent lower than those of conventionally insured populations . . . due almost entirely to lower admission rates. . . . There is no evidence that health maintenance organizations reduce admissions in discretionary or unnecessary categories; rather, the data suggest lower admission rates across the board.

According to Luft, there are three possible interpretations of these data: (1) given that discretionary care exists in all categories of hospitalization, an effective HMO may limit discretionary use across the board; (2) patient self-selection may mean that healthier people, who do not need as much hospitalization, come into HMOs; and (3) HMOs may be skimping at the same time that conventional insurance plans "overtreat" discretionary cases. On the issue of whether or not HMOs provide more health maintenance than conventional insurance plans, Luft (1978b, 163–64) concludes:

> The greater use of preventive services by HMO enrollees appears to be attributable to their better financial coverage, not the preventive care ideology (purported to exist in HMOs). When people have full coverage for 'preventive' ambulatory visits, they have at least as many, if not more, services under the F[ee] F[or] S[ervice] system than in an HMO. These results are entirely in accord with data for hospitalization—HMO enrollees seem to get fewer services if everything else is held constant.

Concerning the ability of HMOs to reduce the growth rate of medical care costs, Luft (1980, 1) concludes that total costs for HMO enrollees since the 1960s "have grown at a slightly lower rate than for people with conventional insurance coverage. Hospitalization rates show substantial reductions within specific HMOs over a 20 year period." Some of the HMOs' long-term reductions in hospitalization, however, may only reflect changes in the age-sex mix of their enrollment populations.

In general terms, these "state-of-the-art" reviews seem to agree on five points (Wolinsky 1980):

1. Hospitalization rates in HMOs are as much as 45 percent lower than those in conventional insurance systems (clearly the case for PGP models, although not so clearly for IPA models).

2. Total costs are less in HMOs than in conventional insurance systems (again, largely because of lower hospitalization rates, and more pronounced in prepaid group practices than in IPA models).

3. Seemingly higher levels of preventive care utilization in HMOs may actually be a reflection of the more extensive coverage that they offer compared with conventional health insurance plans.

4. HMO enrollees tend to be more satisfied with the technical aspects of the medical care that they receive than those in conventional insurance plans, but the conventionally insured are more satisfied with their patient-practitioner relationships.

5. Although the evidence on the quality of care received in HMOs is not complete, that quality appears to be at least equal to, if not better than, that received in the average conventional insurance plans.

Nonetheless, the most important and agreed-upon point to emerge from these reviews is that, although reduced costs and lower hospitalization rates in HMOs are rather well documented, we still do not know how they are achieved.

Identifying the Incentive Bundles
Operative in HMOs

One of the reasons that so little is known about the effects of HMOs on the practice of medicine relates to the definitional problems of what an HMO actually is, the failure to distinguish between some of the basic types of HMOs, and the failure to delineate the general and specific structural incentives and disincentives in HMOs that affect the practice of medicine. Accordingly, a good first step in understanding the promise and performance of HMOs at either the macro or the micro level must begin with a clear definition of what an HMO is. According to Luft (1981), HMOs may best be defined by five essential behavioral characteristics:

— The HMO assumes a contractual responsibility to provide or insure the delivery of a stated range of health services.
— The HMO serves an enrolled, defined population.
— The HMO has a voluntary enrollment of subscribers.
— The HMO requires a fixed periodic payment to the organization that is independent of the use of services.
— The HMO assumes at least part of the financial risk and/or gain in the provision of services.

Contractual responsibility means that HMO members have legal rights to medical care provided by the HMO. In a conventional health care system, physicians have the right to decide whether to take on a new patient. In the HMO, physicians must provide the care that any HMO member needs. Enrolled, defined population means that the HMO knows to whom it is obligated to provide care and can therefore estimate how much care it will need to provide. This allows HMOs to engage in more accurate planning than conventional health care systems. Voluntary enrollment means that enrollees can choose either a conventional plan like Blue Cross/Blue Shield or the HMO. The choice is theirs to make. Fixed periodic payment means that regardless of the number of services used, a given enrollee pays the same predetermined monthly fee. This means that the HMO does not make more money by providing more services, as is the case in the conventional health care system. Finally, financial risk means that the HMO will either financially suffer or benefit from the health care that it delivers.

There are three basic types of HMOs, although within each type there is considerable variation. The three types are group models, staff models, and individual practice associations (IPAs). In a group model HMO, all physicians are members of the same group practice. Their medical group contracts with the HMO to provide its services and is legally and fiscally separate from the HMO. The group usually services the HMO exclusively and either owns or contracts with the hospital to which the patients are admitted. Members of the group are reimbursed on a salary or salary plus profit sharing basis. The key element, then, in group model HMOs is that the physicians have a clear proprietary interest in the success or failure of the group and of the HMO. In essence, they are partners in its financial success or failure. The classic example of group model HMOs is the Kaiser Foundation Health Plan.

Unlike physicians in group models, physicians in staff model HMOs are employed directly by the HMO itself. As a result, they are employees rather than partners. Therefore, they do not have as clear a proprietary interest in the HMO. They are usually reimbursed on a salary basis, although adjustments may be made based on average patient loads. The classic example of a staff model HMO is the Group Health Plan of Puget Sound.

The IPA is a loose federation of independent, individual physicians who agree to treat patients enrolled in a third-party HMO on a fee-for-service basis in their own offices. Frequently the IPA is jointly sponsored by local medical societies and insurance companies. When an IPA physician provides service to an HMO enrollee, the physician is reimbursed by the IPA for services rendered, less a modest allowance for the administration of the plan. Unlike staff and group model physicians who usually have the majority of their patients coming from the HMO, IPA physicians usually have no more than 10 percent of their patients coming from the HMO. As a result, while the HMO practice is usually the major, if not the entire, practice for staff and group model physicians, it is a small sideline for physicians in IPAs. The classic example of an IPA is the Forbes Health Maintenance Plan in Pittsburgh.

According to Wolinsky and Corry (1981), the three major types of HMOs may be differentiated in terms of two key characteristics. These are the organizational constraints embodied in the structure of the HMO itself and the fiscal incentives which affect the physician's behavior. Wolinsky and Corry ignore the constraints and incentives that affect patient behavior, because these are the same in all three HMO types (i.e., moral hazard exists in all HMOs). *Organizational constraints* refer principally to the degree that the various health components in the HMO are structurally integrated into one functional health care system. The more fully integrated the HMO (i.e., the "tighter" the interrelationships between the health care components), the easier it is to implement and supervise standard review processes associated with the practice of medicine. It is also more likely for such standards and procedures to be uniformly applied and result in substantial cost containment as well as modifications of traditional practice patterns.

The *fiscal incentives* that affect HMO physicians reflect whether or not they have a clear proprietary interest in the success or failure of the HMO, as well as the method by which they are reimbursed. The greater the proprietary interest of the physicians, the more likely they are to be conscious of the cost associated with the medical care being provided. Physicians with a clear proprietary interest are more likely to adhere to the cost-containment strategies and, therefore, may be more likely to alter their medical practices from traditional practice patterns.

How the physicians are reimbursed is also very important. Traditionally, physicians have been reimbursed on a fee-for-service basis. Under that arrangement the incentive facing physicians is to provide more services (or to substitute more expensive services), because providing more (or more expensive) services generates more (or higher) fees. Thus, the fee-for-service system contains the potentially perverse incentive for physicians to provide more (or more costly) services than their patients actually need. The alternative to the fee-for-service system used in group and staff model HMOs is the capitation-based system. Under that arrangement, physicians are reimbursed by essentially a flat rate per patient, regardless of the amount or kind of services provided. On the one hand, this eliminates the incentive to provide more (or more expensive) services than their patients actually need. On the other hand, it creates the new and potentially perverse incentive for physicians to provide fewer services (or to substitute less expensive services) than their patients actually need. Thus, physicians who are reimbursed on a fee-for-service basis may be more likely to overprovide (or substitute more expensive services), while their prepaid counterparts may be more likely to underprovide (or substitute less expensive services).

Table 1.1 summarizes Wolinsky and Corry's (1981) conceptual model. Physicians in IPAs have low levels on both the organizational constraints and the fiscal incentives (i.e., they do not practice out of a well-integrated health care delivery system, and they are reimbursed on a fee-for-service basis). Therefore, it is expected that their medical practices would be most like those of physicians in the traditional fee-for-service, unintegrated health care delivery system. Physicians in staff model HMOs are subject to a low level of fiscal incentives, combined with a high level of organizational constraints (i.e., although they work within a capitation-based, integrated system, they do not have strong proprietary interests in that system). Thus, their medical practices are expected to be somewhat different from those of physicians in either IPAs or in the conventional fee-for-service health care delivery system. Finally, group model HMO physicians have high levels of both organizational constraints and fiscal incentives (i.e., they work in a capitation-based, integrated system in which they have strong proprietary interests). Their medical practices are most likely to be different from those of physicians in the conventional fee-for-service system. In addition, their medical practices are also expected to be different from those of either IPA or staff model HMO physicians.

Figure 1.4 graphically portrays the approximate expected relative differences in the practice of medicine for the three types of HMOs and for solo and group fee-for-service practices, based on the Wolinsky and Corry (1981) model. The reader should note that although the continuum shown in figure 1.4 (and subsequently in figure 1.5) appears to be unidimensional, it represents the combina-

Table 1.1   Levels of organizational con-
            straints (i.e., system integration)
            and fiscal incentives (i.e., pro-
            prietary interest) by type of HMO

HMO Type	Organizational Constraints	Fiscal Incentives
IPA model	Low	Low
Staff model	High	Low
Group model	High	High

Source: F. Wolinsky and B. Corry, "Organizational Structure and
Medical Practice in Health Maintenance Organizations," in *Pro-
file of Medical Practice, 1981,* edited by D. Goldfarb. Chicago:
American Medical Association, 1981. Reprinted with permission.

tion of the organizational constraints and fiscal incentives described above. As
figure 1.4 indicates, one would expect a considerable difference between the practice of medicine in solo fee-for-service settings and in group fee-for-service settings. (The literature demonstrating these differences has been reviewed above.)
The differences between the IPA model HMO and group fee-for-service practices, however, are expected to be very small, if observable at all. This is because
the organizational constraints and a low level of fiscal incentives in IPA model
HMO and group fee-for-service practices are essentially identical. The group model
HMO, however, is expected to be at the other end of the continuum, because
it represents high levels of both organizational constraints and fiscal incentives.
The staff model HMO falls somewhere between the group model HMO and group
fee-for-service practice settings, because it contains a high level of organizational
constraints and a low level of fiscal incentives. Accordingly, the Wolinsky and
Corry typology suggests that in evaluating the effect of HMOs on the practice
of medicine, the particular type of HMO under investigation must be taken into
consideration.

More recently, Luft (1983) has taken the conceptual and methodological
issues concerning the evaluation of the effect of HMOs on the practice of medicine
one step further. With regard to the methodological issues, Luft (1983, 321–22)
suggests four very important cautionary notes that must be considered:

The *first* stems from the diversity of HMOs. To understand the published findings,
one must view each HMO as a unique entity. Yet to be useful for policy makers,
results must be generalizable, and thus the findings of multiple studies may have
to be combined. . . . The *second* caution relates to the data available for analysis.
A recent comprehensive review of the published evidence on HMO performance
indicates that available data vary in depth, breadth, and quality (i.e., reliability and
validity). . . . The *third* caution relates to the source of published findings on HMO
performance. The vast majority of the existing findings relate to a handful of large,

well established plans. . . . Research on these mature HMOs may not be directly applicable to new, developing plans. *Fourth*, there have been no randomized, controlled experiments that involve the assignment of a representative group of people to a wide range of health maintenance organizations and traditional health insurance plans. . . . Therefore, while we can say that cost (or utilization, or satisfaction) are lower in one situation than another, we cannot determine if the differences are attributable to general characteristics of the plans, to unique features of the providers and administrators, or to subtle differences among the people selecting the plan, that is the potential for self-selection.

Luft goes on to suggest that because HMOs have been touted as one of the leading remedies for the ills in the health care delivery system, more detailed and exacting evaluations of HMO performance are needed.

In calling for additional research on the effect of HMOs on the practice of medicine, Luft (1983) argues that such new studies must take into consideration the two leading factors that influence how a particular HMO "develops, grows, and performs": internal organizational characteristics of the plan and environmental characteristics related to the plan's location. With regard to the internal organizational factors, Luft identifies six crucial areas: (1) sponsorship and goals; (2) organizational and administrative structure; (3) method of paying the physicians; (4) physician staffing; (5) control of hospital services; and (6) marketing of services. The sponsorship and goals factors are essentially an analog to the same issues in extant discussions of hospital performance (private versus public, forprofit versus not-for-profit, religious versus nonreligious). The organizational and administrative structure issues are remarkably similar to the system integration factors described by Wolinsky and Corry (1981). The method of paying the physicians is divided into three basic approaches: fee-for-service, straight salary, and capitation arrangements. To some extent, the physician reimbursement issue is an analog of the physician incentives also described by Wolinsky and Corry. Physician staffing issues refer to the size, specialty mix, and full- or part-time participation of physicians in the plans. The control of hospital services issue focuses on whether or not the HMO has its own hospital facility, whether it contracts on a long-term basis with local facilities, or whether it obtains services as needed at prevailing rates within the community. Finally, the marketing of services issue

Figure 1.4   Approximate expected relative differences in the practice of medicine between the three types of HMOs and solo and group fee-for-service practices

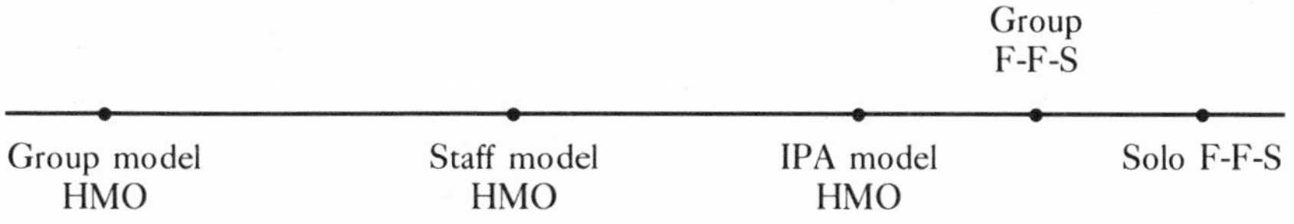

		Group F-F-S	
Group model HMO	Staff model HMO	IPA model HMO	Solo F-F-S

treats the aggressive nature of the sales staff associated with the HMO, as well as its federal qualification status (which mandates that the HMO be offered in dual-choice situations within the immediate geographic area).

The external factors that Luft identifies are in two categories: local sociodemographic market characteristics and regulatory requirements. With regard to the local sociodemographic market characteristics, Luft points out that some HMOs are more attractive to certain types of people than others. Accordingly, in areas where the population might have an "affinity" for a certain type of HMO, that HMO may be more successful, both in terms of enrollment and cost containment. Similarly, in some areal marketplaces health benefit packages may be more or less advantageous for the HMO. Also, "bandwagon" effects may be associated with HMO growth and performance in areas where market penetration begins to reach appreciable levels.

Regulatory requirements focus more on the issue of whether the HMO is forced to operate at a competitive disadvantage with conventional health insurance plans because of requirements established under the state HMO enabling acts or under the federal HMO Act of 1973. For example, some states require very extensive audits of utilization and quality assurance data in order to monitor HMO performance, while other states take a far less regulatory approach to HMOs. Similarly, in some states the HMO legislation does not mandate adequate protection for plan enrollees if the HMO fails (although all states mandate such protection arrangements for non-HMO insured persons). Thus, in some states joining an HMO involves more risk than in other states.

One additional factor that has not been explicitly addressed by either Luft (1983) or Wolinsky and Corry (1981) is the recent appearance of "hybrid" group model HMOs. That is, in the past several years a number of group practices that were basically fee-for-service arrangements have begun to offer their services on a prepaid basis in order to enhance their areal market position. Krill and Gaynor (1982) have labeled these new hybrid model HMOs "FFS/PPD" groups, indicating the mix of fee-for-service and prepaid practice. Although the FFS/PPD designation has not been widely adopted in the literature, the importance of the distinction between the "traditional" Kaiser-brand group model HMOs and the "hybrid" group model HMOs is important (see Wolinsky and Marder 1982a). The crucial sociological and economic distinctions between the hybrids and the traditional Kaiser group model HMOs turn on the fact that in the Kaiser model HMOs all of the participating physicians' practices consist entirely of prepaid patients; in the hybrid model HMOs the participating physicians' practices are only partially composed of prepaid patients. Moreover, during the early years of a hybrid group model HMO, the percentage of prepaid patients seen by the participating physicians is likely to be small, because penetration of the prepaid market historically involves a slow, developmental process. Accordingly, although there is not yet a precise method by which to differentiate how closely the hybrid group model

HMOs approximate the traditional Kaiser model HMOs, a simplistic distinction between the two forms of group model HMOs can and should be made.

When taken collectively, the works of Freidson (1970), Wolinsky and Corry (1981), Luft (1983), and Krill and Gaynor (1982) suggest that there are at least six viable distinctions among and between the practice settings in which physicians currently may practice medicine in the United States. Among the fee-for-service practice settings, there are the traditional solo and group practices. Among the prepaid practice settings, there are the traditional Kaiser group model HMOs, the hybrid non-Kaiser group model HMOs, the staff model HMOs, and the IPAs (although the latter may actually beg the question of what actually is prepaid, at least beyond the patient's perspective).

Figure 1.5 portrays the ordering and approximate relative placement of the six practice settings on the autonomous-bureaucratic continuum of medical practice (based on organizational constraints and fiscal incentives) that underlies most discussions of the organization of medical practice. As indicated in figure 1.5, going from the autonomous to the bureaucratic end of the continuum (i.e., from right to left), one encounters solo fee-for-service practices, group fee-for-service practices, IPA model HMOs, staff model HMOs, non-Kaiser group model HMOs, and Kaiser group model HMOs. The letters above the distances between any two contiguous practice settings in figure 1.5 are used to simplify our discussion of the relative distances between practice settings on the autonomous–bureaucratic dimension of medical practice.

The letter *a* represents the distance between solo and group fee-for-service settings. As discussed earlier, there are significant differences in the personal autonomy of a physician in these two practice settings, and there are differences in the way that medicine is practiced between these two settings. The letter *b* represents the difference between group fee-for-service settings and the IPA model HMO. According to our theory, the difference (i.e., the distance) represented

Figure 1.5 **Ordering and approximate relative placement of the six practice settings on the autonomous-bureaucratic continuum of medical practice**

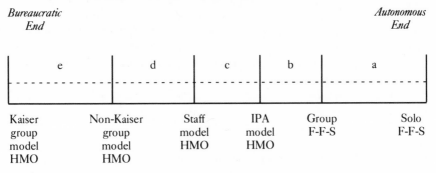

Bureaucratic End

Autonomous End

e	d	c	b	a
Kaiser group model HMO	Non-Kaiser group model HMO	Staff model HMO	IPA model HMO	Group F-F-S	Solo F-F-S

by *b* is inconsequential. That is, our theory postulates that there are no significant differences in the practice of medicine in group fee-for-service settings compared with IPA model HMOs. The distance on the autonomous–bureaucratic
dimension of medical practice between IPA model HMOs (or for that matter,
group fee-for-service settings, as no meaningful distance separates these two practice settings) and staff model HMOs (depicted by the letter *c*), non-Kaiser group
model HMOs (*c* plus *d*), and Kaiser group model HMOs (*c* plus *d* plus *e*) are quite
significant in our theory. That is, we expect the practice of medicine in staff model
HMOs to be different from that in either IPA model HMOs or group fee-for-
service practices. Similarly, we predict that the practice of medicine in non-Kaiser
group model HMOs will also be different, but that it will, in addition, be different
from that in staff model HMOs. Finally, we predict that the practice of medicine
in Kaiser group model HMOs will be different from that in all of the preceding
practice settings.

These differences, with one exception, are those discussed earlier in
reference to the conceptual model of Wolinsky and Corry (1981). The one exception is as follows. At present, the literature is not sufficiently well developed to
precisely specify the relative differences on the autonomous-bureaucratic dimension of medical practice between staff model HMOs, non-Kaiser group model
HMOs, and Kaiser group model HMOs. That is, although the literature is sufficiently well developed to specify that *d* and *e* are significantly different from zero,
we are not yet in a position to speculate on the magnitude of *d* relative to *e*, or
to *c*, or to *a*. Nonetheless, the conceptual model of the settings in which medicine
may be practiced does allow us to specify the relative ordering of the six practice
settings along the autonomous-bureaucratic continuum. Therefore, this portion
of the conceptual framework can be submitted to empirical verification.

Remaining Issues and the
General Analytic Model

The previous sections of this chapter began with Freidson's conceptual model
of the organization of medical practice and brought it into the 1980s by summariz-
ing several recent and newly emergent practice settings. Based on that conceptual framework, we now formalize the general analytic model that guides this study,
address the remaining issues concerning the data used to test that model, and
present the plan for the remaining chapters.

The general analytic model derived from the conceptual framework described
above is shown in its functional form in equation 1:

$$POM = f(SD, EN, AT, PS) \qquad (1)$$

where *POM* refers to the practice of medicine, *f* denotes that the practice of
medicine is a function of the characteristics shown in the following parenthetical

statement, *SD* represents the sociodemographic characteristics of the physician, *EN* represents the environmental characteristics that may either constrain or enhance a physician's opportunity to practice medicine, *AT* represents the attitudinal characteristics indicative of the physician's preference structure (reflecting upon the self-selection issue), and *PS* represents the practice setting in which the physician works (solo fee-for-service, group fee-for-service, IPA model HMOs, staff model HMOs, non-Kaiser group model HMOs, or Kaiser group model HMOs).

Note that there are no subscripts in equation 1. In a perfectly specified model defining the practice of medicine, there would be two subscripts for each term in the function defined in equation 1. That is, the effect of the sociodemographic (*SD*) characteristics on the practice of medicine would be subscripted for both the patient and the practitioner. The same would be true for the environmental (*EN*) characteristics, the attitudinal (*AT*) characteristics, and the practice settings (*PS*) characteristics. Thus, in a perfectly specified model, the practice of medicine would be defined as a function of the sociodemographic, environmental, attitudinal, and practice setting characteristics of both the physician and the patient. (See Hooper et al. 1982 for a discussion of patient characteristics that affect physician behavior.) Although we clearly recognize that the terms in equation 1 should be doubly subscripted, we have not done so because of the awesome difficulties involved in collecting such detailed information on both physicians and their patients at the same time. Indeed, it is difficult enough to find a data set with sufficiently detailed information on either patients *or* their physicians. Accordingly, we have presented the general analytic model in its simplistic form (i.e., from just the physician's perspective).

Having identified the difficulties of obtaining such information simultaneously on physicians and patients, we now submit that for at least two of the four sets of terms in equation 1 (the *SD, EN, AT,* and *PS* terms), the values for the patient and the practitioner are likely to be similar, if not identical. The value of the environmental characteristics (*EN*) and the practice setting (*PS*) will likely be the same for both the patient and the physician. This is most obvious for the practice setting, which will be the same for the patient and the physician in any particular patient-practitioner interaction. The environmental characteristics should also be comparable for both the patient and the physician, although the true, areal marketplaces for the two may not completely overlap. Accordingly, although we have described the four terms in equation 1 from the perspective of the physician, we believe that the effects of the environmental characteristics and the practice setting from the patient's perspective are sufficiently congruent with those from the physician's perspective so as not to seriously jeopardize the specification of the general analytic model by their absence.

The absence in equation 1 of the patient's sociodemographic and attitudinal characteristics, however, is another matter. It could reasonably be argued that the attitudinal characteristics of the patient (especially with regard to the self-selection issue) are likely to be consonant with those of the physician, under the assumption that there is an affinity between patients and physicians concerning their attitudes and perspectives on matters medical. (See Ross, Wheaton, and Duff 1981 for an insightful discussion of this issue, and Wolinsky and Steiber 1982 for a review of the literature on how patients select their physicians; both studies support this assumption.) It is not at all straightforward, however, to assume that the sociodemographic characteristics of patients are consonant with those of their physicians. Thus, if equation 1 is estimated using data only from the physician's perspective, at least one term (SD) will remain essentially unobserved from the patient's perspective.

There are, then, two issues that remain to be addressed. First, what will be the effect of not incorporating data from the patient's perspective (i.e., what will be lost) in assessing the effects of practice settings on the practice of medicine? Unfortunately, this is an empirical question that cannot be addressed given our present knowledge. It can be said, however, that all extant assessments of the effect of practice settings on the practice of medicine (e.g., the literature reviewed earlier on the differences between solo and group practice settings) have *not* contained any direct measures from the patient's perspective regarding the terms identified in equation 1. Although this certainly does not justify the omission of data from the patient's perspective, it does demonstrate that the present study will, no less than previous studies, incorporate data from the patient's perspective. Thus, although the absence of data from the patient's perspective limits the precision with which we can evaluate the general analytic model expressed in equation 1, our study is no more limited in this respect than previous studies.

Second, what contribution can the empirical assessment of the general analytic model expressed in equation 1 provide, based solely on data from the physician's perspective? In our view, the answer to this question is the ability to assess the impact of both the organization of medical practice on the practice of medicine net of the sociodemographic and environmental characteristics of the physician and the attitudinal characteristics which might have led different physicians to select different practice settings. That is, this general analytic model permits us to partition out, to a degree, the self-selection issue, and to partition out the traditional sociodemographic and environmental characteristics from the "true" net effects of practice setting on the practice of medicine. In so doing, we will be able not only to separate the nature effects from the nurture effects; we will also be able to compare the relative importance of the nature effects and the nurture effects, as well as the traditional control factors (i.e., the sociodemographic and environmental characteristics of the physician). In conjunction with our six-fold typology of practice settings, then, these are the contributions that this general analytic model should permit us to make to the growing literature on the effect of the organization of medical practice on the practice of medicine.

In order to assess this general analytic model, we rely on data taken from the fourteenth Periodic Survey of Physicians (PSP–14) conducted by the AMA

Center for Health Services Research and Development in 1980. These data are generally well known in the literature and are described in great detail in chapter 2. The PSP–14 data allow us to fully assess the general analytic model's ability to predict a variety of indicators of the practice of medicine, including patient queues, the amount of time that physicians spend with their patients, physician incomes and expenses, and so forth. Indeed, in several previous papers we have used these same PSP–14 data to begin the exploration of the effects of the organization of medical practice on the practice of medicine (see Wolinsky and Marder 1982b, 1983a, 1983b). The present study will, for the very first time, use these data to assess the complete general analytic model shown in equation 1.

The remainder of this monograph is divided into four chapters. Chapter 2 presents and reviews the PSP–14 data that are used to assess the general analytic model expressed in equation 1. Chapter 3 presents the results of applying the general analytic model to data on the practice of medicine from the patient's perspective. In particular, the focus there is on the net effects of the organization of medical practice on patient queues and on the amount of time that physicians spend with their patients. Chapter 4 presents the results of applying the general analytic model to various aspects of the practice of medicine from the physician's perspective. In particular, it examines the net effect of the organization of medical practice on physician workloads, incomes, and professional expenses. Finally, chapter 5 reviews the success of the typology of the organization of medical practice presented in this chapter with the results presented in chapters 3 and 4. Suggested modifications of the new typology are discussed at that point, as are the implications of the results and of the new typology for the future of the health care delivery system in the United States.

References

Berkanovic, Emil; Carol Telesky; and Sharon Reeder. 1981. "Structural and social psychological factors in the decision to seek medical care for symptoms." *Medical Care* 19:693–709.

Berki, Sylvester, and Marie Ashcraft. 1980. "HMO enrollment: Who joins what and why: A review of the literature." *Milbank Memorial Fund Quarterly* 58:588–632.

Breslau, Naomi; Geritt Wolf; and Alvin Novack. 1978a. "Correlates of physicians' task delegation in primary care." *Journal of Health and Social Behavior* 19:374–84.

Breslau, Naomi; Alvin Novack; and Gerritt Wolf. 1978b. "Work settings and job satisfaction: A study of primary care physicians and paramedical personnel." *Medical Care* 16:850–62.

Burkett, Gary. 1982. "Variations in physician utilization patterns in a capitation payment IPA–HMO." *Medical Care* 20:1128–39.

Department of Health, Education, and Welfare. 1974. *Federal Register*, Vol. 38, No. 203. Washington, D.C.: Government Printing Office.

_____. 1975. *Health Maintenance Organizations: Guides for Subparts B, C, D, E, and G.* Washington, D.C.: Government Printing Office.

Donabedian, Avedis. 1969. "An evaluation of prepaid group practice." *Inquiry* 6:3–27.

Dutton, Diana. 1979. "Patterns of ambulatory health care in five different delivery systems." *Medical Care* 17:221–39.

Eisenberg, John. 1979. "Sociologic influences on decision-making by clinicians." *Annals of Internal Medicine* 90:957–64.

Eisenberg, John; Anita Mackie; Lawrence Kahn; and Gerald Perkoff. 1974. "Patterns of pediatric practice by the same physicians in a prepaid and a fee-for-service setting." *Clinical Pediatrics* 13:352–59.

Ellwood, Paul. 1971. "Health maintenance organizations: Concepts and strategy." *Hospitals* 45:53–56.

Freidson, Eliot. 1970. *Profession of medicine: A study of the sociology of applied knowledge.* New York: Harper and Row.

Freshnock, Larry, and Louis Goodman. 1979. "Medical group practice in the United States: Patterns of survival between 1969 and 1975." *Journal of Health and Social Behavior* 20:352–62.

_____. 1980. "The organization of physician services in solo and group medical practice." *Medical Care* 18:17–29.

Gaus, Clifton; Barbara Cooper; and C. Hirschman. 1976. "Contrasts in HMO and fee-for-service performance." *Social Security Bulletin* 39:3–14.

Goodman, Louis, and James Swartwout. 1984. "Comparative aspects of medical practice: Organizational setting and financial arrangements in four delivery systems." *Medical Care* 22:255–66.

Goodman, Louis, and Fredric Wolinsky. 1982. "Conditional logit analysis of physicians' practice mode choices." *Inquiry* 19:262–70.

Graham, Fred. 1972. "Group versus solo practice: Arguments and evidence." *Inquiry* 9:49–60.

Gray, Lois. 1980. "Consumer satisfaction with physician provided services: A panel study." *Social Science and Medicine* 14A:65–73.

Greenley, James, and Stuart Kirk. 1976. "Organizational influences on access to health care." *Social Science and Medicine* 10:317–22.

Greenlick, Merwynn. 1972. "The impact of prepaid group practice on American medical care: A critical evaluation." *Annals of the American Academy of Political and Social Science* 399:100–113.

Hall, Oswald. 1946. "The informal organization of the medical profession." *Canadian Journal of Economics and Political Science* 12:30–41.

_____. 1949. "Types of medical careers." *American Journal of Sociology* 55:243–53.

Hooper, Elizabeth; Loretto Comstock; Jean Goodwin; and James Goodwin. 1982. "Patient characteristics that influence physician behavior." *Medical Care* 20:630–37.

Hull, J. 1979. "Factors influencing styles of medical practice: The use of psychiatric referrals by non-psychiatric physicians." *Medical Care* 17:718–26.

Klarman, Herbert. 1963. "The effects of prepaid group practice on hospital use." *Public Health Reports* 78:955–65.

Krill, Mary, and Ralph Gaynor. 1982. "An assessment of the future of HMOs." *Medical Group Management* 29:42–46.

Levine, Sol; Jacob Feldman; and Jack Elinson. 1983. "Does medical care do any good?" In *Handbook of Health, Health Care, and the Health Professions*, edited by David Mechanic. New York: Free Press.

Luft, Harold. 1978a. "How do health maintenance organizations achieve their savings? Rhetoric and evidence." *New England Journal of Medicine* 298:1336–43.

———. 1978b. "Why do HMOs seem to provide more health maintenance services?" *Milbank Memorial Fund Quarterly* 56:140–68.

———. 1979. "HMOs, competition, cost containment, and NHI." Paper presented at the meetings of the American Enterprise Institute, Washington, D.C.

———. 1980. "Trends in medical care costs: Do HMOs lower the rate of growth?" *Medical Care* 18:1–16.

———. 1981. *Health Maintenance Organizations: Dimensions of Performance*. New York: Wiley.

———. 1983. "Health maintenance organizations." In *Handbook of Health, Health Care, and the Health Professions*, edited by David Mechanic. New York: Free Press.

Luke, Roice, and Michael Thomson. 1980a. "Utilization of within-hospital services: A study of the effects of two forms of group practice." *Medical Care* 18:219–27.

———. 1980b. "Group practice affiliation and interphysician consulting patterns within a community general hospital." *Journal of Health and Social Behavior* 21: 334–44.

Mahoney, Anne. 1973. "Factors affecting physicians' choice of group or independent practice." *Inquiry* 10:9–18.

McElrath, Donald. 1961. "Perspective and participation of physicians in prepaid group practice." *American Sociological Review* 26:596–608.

Mechanic, David. 1975. "The organization of medical practice and practice orientations among physicians in prepaid and nonprepaid primary care settings." *Medical Care* 13:189–204.

Mick, Stephen et al. 1983. "Physician turnover in eight New England prepaid group practices: An analysis." *Medical Care* 21:323–37.

Nixon, Richard. 1971. *Health Message of the President of the United States*. Washington, D.C.: Government Printing Office.

Perkoff, Gerald. 1978. "An effect of organization of medical care upon health manpower distribution." *Medical Care* 8:628–40.

PL 93–222. 1973. *The Health Maintenance Organization Act of 1973*. Washington, D.C.: Government Printing Office.

PL 93–641. 1974. *The National Health Planning and Resources Development Act of 1974*. Washington, D.C.: Government Printing Office.

PL 94–460. 1976. *Health Maintenance Organization Amendments of 1976*. Washington, D.C.: Government Printing Office.

PL 95–559. 1978. *Health Maintenance Organization Amendments of 1978*. Washington, D.C.: Government Printing Office.

Rhee, Sang-O. 1977. "Relative importance of physicians' personal and situational characteristics for the quality of patient care." *Journal of Health and Social Behavior* 18:10–15.

Rhee, Sang-O; Roice Luke; and Melissa Culverwell. 1980. "Influence of client/colleague dependence on physician performance in patient care." *Medical Care* 18:829–39.

Roemer, Milton, and William Shonick. 1973. "HMO performance: The recent evidence." *Milbank Memorial Fund Quarterly* 51:271–317.

Roos, Noralou. 1980. "Impact of the organization of practice on quality of care and physician productivity." *Medical Care* 18:347–59.

Ross, Catherine, and Raymond Duff. 1982. "Returning to the doctor: The effect of client characteristics, type of practice, and experiences with care." *Journal of Health and Social Behavior* 23:11–31.

Ross, Catherine; John Mirowsky; and Raymond Duff. 1982. "Physician status characteristics and client satisfaction in two types of medical practice." *Journal of Health and Social Behavior* 23:317–29.

Ross, Catherine; Blair Wheaton; and Raymond Duff. 1981. "Client satisfaction and the organization of medical practice: Why time counts." *Journal of Health and Social Behavior* 22:243–55.

Shortell, Stephen. 1972. *A Model of Physician Referral Behavior: A Test of Exchange Theory in Practice.* Chicago: Center for Health Administration Studies.

Shortell, Stephen et al. 1977. "The relationships among dimensions of health services in two provider systems: A causal model approach." *Journal of Health and Social Behavior* 18:139–59.

Surgeon General. 1979. *Healthy People: The Surgeon General's Report on Health Promotion and Disease Prevention.* Publication Number 79–55071. Washington, D.C.: Government Printing Office.

Tessler, Richard, and David Mechanic. 1976. "Consumer satisfaction with prepaid group practice: A comparative study." *Journal of Health and Social Behavior* 14:95–113.

Weinerman, Edward. 1964. "Patients' perceptions of group medical care: A review and analysis of studies of choice and utilization of prepaid group practice plans." *American Journal of Public Health* 54:880–89.

Williamson, P. M. 1975. "The adoption of new drugs by doctors practicing in group and solo practice." *Social Science and Medicine* 9:233–36.

Wolinsky, Fredric. 1980. "The performance of health maintenance organizations: An analytic review." *Milbank Memorial Fund Quarterly* 58:537–82.

———. 1982. "Why physicians choose different types of practice settings." *Health Services Research* 17:399–419.

Wolinsky, Fredric, and Barbara Corry. 1981. "Organizational structure and medical practice in health maintenance organizations." In *Profile of Medical Practice, 1981,* edited by David Goldfarb. Chicago: American Medical Association.

Wolinsky, Fredric, and William Marder. 1982a. "HMOs: The concept, new evidence and implications." *Medical Group Management* 29:50–52, 58.

———. 1982b. "Spending time with patients: The impact of organizational structure on medical practice." *Medical Care* 20:1051–59.

———. 1983a. "Waiting to see the doctor: The impact of organizational structure on medical practice." *Medical Care* 21:531–42.

———. 1983b. "The organization of medical practice and primary care physician income." *American Journal of Public Health* 73:379–82.

Wolinsky, Fredric, and Steven Steiber. 1982. "Salient issues in choosing a new doctor." *Social Science and Medicine* 16:759–67.

2

Using the Periodic Survey
of Physicians to Assess
the General Analytic Model

Overview

The purpose of this chapter is fourfold. First, we review the history and method of data collection involved in the American Medical Association's Periodic Survey of Physicians. Second, we examine the reliability and validity of the data obtained from the Periodic Survey of Physicians, with special regard to its suitability for assessing the effects of the organization of medical practice on the practice of medicine. Third, we describe in detail the two Periodic Surveys of Physicians that serve as the data base for this study. Finally, we present some basic cross-tabular analyses of various aspects of the practice of medicine by the organizational settings in which they occur, as well as some data on the self-selection issue.

History of the Periodic Survey
of Physicians

The American Medical Association (AMA) maintains a data base consisting of current and historical information on every known physician in the United States, regardless of membership in the AMA, including American medical graduates who are practicing abroad as well as foreign medical graduates practicing within the United States. This data base is referred to as the "Masterfile" and has been shown in numerous studies to be highly reliable and accurate when compared with data obtained from a variety of other sources. Indeed, with respect to physician location information the Masterfile is accurate within a range of 2 to 6.6 percent (see Goodman and Eisenberg 1977).

The Masterfile is generally considered the authoritative data base on physicians in the United States, and all federal physician manpower estimates are derived from it (cf. Jensen, Wunderman, and Goodman 1982). It is so accurate and highly regarded because of its computerized data entry system which continuously updates the validity and completeness of the information on the physicians. According to Goodman and Jensen (1981), about 3,000 physician updates are triggered and processed each week as a result of routine AMA mailings, correspondence with physicians, and communications with other public and private organizations. In addition, a triennial census of all physicians is conducted, and that information is incorporated into the Masterfile.

Although the Masterfile is an almost impeccable data base, it is not without limitations. Two of these have serious implications for using the Masterfile in health services research. First, although the basic demographic data are highly reliable and valid, characteristics monitoring the physician's professional activity are not so accurate. Second, given that the Masterfile is an enumeration of all physicians, it becomes prohibitively expensive to obtain more detailed data on the practice of medicine using this format. Accordingly, in the mid–1960s the Center for Health Services Research and Development of the AMA began to design the Periodic Survey of Physicians (PSP) to augment the Masterfile. Theodore and Sutter (1966) described the purpose of the PSP as fourfold: (1) comparing data from the Masterfile with data from the PSP on specialty and professional activity variables, (2) developing a descriptive profile of the physician population, (3) estimating a variety of characteristics concerning the practice of medicine, including the number of weeks worked per year, the number of hours practiced per week, and the number of patients seen, and (4) assessing the feasibility of having surveys, such as the PSP, conducted in-house by the AMA.

Beginning with the first PSP survey conducted in 1966, the basic design has always relied upon a representative sample of office-based physicians engaged in active medical practice in the United States. To produce such a representative group of office-based physicians, a probability sample is first selected from the Masterfile. For the most recent of the PSP surveys, the sampling technique has been a stratified systematic probability sample of about 5 percent of all nonfederal, office-based physicians practicing in the United States. Proportional stratification is based upon a nine-category classification of medical specialty, including general or family practice, internal medicine, surgery, pediatrics, obstetrics/gynecology, radiology, psychiatry, anesthesiology, and other specialties. The size of the PSP sample has historically depended upon both the desired precision of the population estimates to be obtained and the expected response rates.

The PSP survey instrument is printed on the front and back of one double-sized sheet of paper folded to provide four pages. A facsimile of the PSP questionnaire used in 1980 is found in the Appendix. The first page of the PSP instrument is a cover letter from the executive vice president of the AMA explaining the purpose of the survey, assuring confidentiality of the data provided, and requesting each physician's participation. The three remaining pages are devoted to close-ended or precoded questions that may be divided into two categories. The first category of questions is the "core" section, which is subject to only the most minor revisions from year to year in order to maintain the integrity of time line or trend analyses. The core section solicits detailed data on practice setting characteristics, the number of hours practiced and patients seen, and professional incomes and expenses. The second component of questions is the "research" section, which may vary substantially from one PSP to another depending upon the specific objectives in the research program of the Center for Health Services Research and Development at the AMA. The research section has recently solicited detailed data on practice settings and variations in reimbursement structures.

Confidentiality of physician responses is maintained in the following manner. First, the PSP sample is drawn from the Masterfile. Second, a four-character alphanumeric identifier is computer-printed on a PSP questionnaire with the name and address of each physician selected for the PSP sample. The physician's name and address are printed on a perforated section of the PSP questionnaire that may be easily detached by the physician. Third, the PSP questionnaires are mailed out, and follow-up questionnaires are sent to nonresponders after about a month, a process which is usually repeated four times. Fourth, the Center for Health Services Research and Development, which receives the completed PSP questionnaires, codes and forwards them to the AMA computer center, where they are keypunched and linked to both the Masterfile and the Area Resources File (ARF). The ARF file, which is available for public use, is prepared by the Bureau of Health Professions (Department of Health and Human Services) and contains a variety of data aggregated at the county level (e.g., hospital bed to population ratios, family income levels, and the like). Finally, a linked file in which all personal identifiers have been removed is returned to the AMA's Center for Health Services Research and Development for analysis.

Although somewhat awkward, this system maximizes confidentiality while permitting the monthly follow-up mailings to be sent to the nonresponding physicians. The four-character alphanumeric linkage file is updated every week of the survey with regard to whether a physician has responded to the questionnaire. This ensures that physicians do not continue to receive PSP questionnaires after they have responded; it also enables accurate response rates to be calculated at the end of the survey.

As indicated, in addition to the initial mailing of the PSP survey instrument to the selected sample of physicians, a number of follow-up mailings and other reminders have been used to increase the response rate. In general, nonresponding physicians have been sent four or five follow-up questionnaires or "telegram-like" messages requesting that they respond to the survey. (In some PSP surveys, telephone follow-ups have been tried on an experimental basis; see Goodman and Jensen 1981.) In the first PSP survey, a response rate of approximately 80 percent was achieved with the original mailing of the questionnaire and three follow-up mailings of questionnaires at approximately monthly intervals.

As indicated by the data in table 2.1, however, the PSP survey response rate declined to about 50 percent by the mid–1970s and has remained stable at that level through 1980. It is generally assumed that the decline in the response rate to the PSP surveys is a result of an increasing hesitation by the American public in general and physicians in particular to provide organizations with such personal information. Another factor has been the marked increase in the number of surveys directed at physicians. To counter the trend in declining response rates, a number of experiments were devised by the AMA Center for Health Services Research and Development. In general, however, these have not been successful (see Goodman and Jensen 1981). As a result, the response rate to the PSP survey has remained at about the 50 percent level when four follow-up questionnaires and a "telegram-like" reminder are used (for a total of six mailings).

Reliability and Validity of the PSP Data

Using the data derived from the PSP surveys for analytical purposes assumes that they are both reliable and valid. Although a variety of statistical techniques exist to assess the reliability of various measures, most of these are not directly applicable to data obtained from the PSP surveys. This is because most reliability assessment techniques concentrate on demonstrating internal consistency among a scale of items tapping the same dimension or upon test-retest stability in responses to questions over a short period of time during which "true" changes are not likely to have occurred (cf. Carmines and Zeller 1979). The question format typically used in the PSP survey, however, does not employ multiple item scales. Rather, single items or questions are used to tap different dimensions of physicians' practice patterns. Moreover, once physicians have responded to a PSP survey instrument they are not recontacted; they are specifically excluded from possible selection for the next two PSP surveys. Accordingly, test-retest reliability estimation procedures are also inappropriate for use with the PSP survey data.

There are, however, other indirect methods of assessing the reliability of the data obtained in the PSP surveys. In particular, members of the AMA Center for Health Services Research and Development have written several papers chronicling a particular practice characteristic over a particular decade. For example, Glandon and Werner (1980) examined both the real and nominal net income reported by physicians responding to the PSP surveys during the 1970s. They found that the real income of physicians remained constant over this period and

Table 2.1   The PSP surveys, sample sizes, and response rates

PSP Number	Year Data Based On	Year Data Collected	Usable Sample Size	Response Rate	Number of Mailings
1	1966	1967	2,833	79.9	4
2	1967	1968	3,704	70.4	5
3	1968	1969	4,125	70.1	6
4	1969	1970	3,449	68.3	4
5	1970	1971	4,689	62.0	4
6	1971	1972	5,020	64.0	4
7	1972	1973	5,085	55.5	6
8	1973	1974	4,195	55.9	5
9	1974	1975	5,016	48.7	4
10	1975	1976	5,288	51.4	5
11	1976	1977	5,330	50.0	5
12	1977	1978	4,455	48.7	6
13	1978	1979	4,506	50.8	6
14	1979	1980	5,133	50.3	6

Source: Adapted from L. Goodman and L. Jensen, "The American Medical Association's Periodic Survey of Physicians." In *Profile of Medical Practice, 1981,* edited by D. Goldfarb. Chicago: American Medical Association, 1981. Reprinted with permission.

that the self-reported nominal income of physicians rose consistently with the general increase in the cost of living. Similarly, other AMA researchers have documented either a remarkable consistency or changes in predicted directions in the average number of hours worked per week, patient visits per week, or number of hours spent with patients in the hospital and in the office when various PSP surveys are compared with each other (cf. Glandon and Shapiro 1980a, 1980b, 1980c). Accordingly, although no direct assessments of the reliability of the PSP survey data have been conducted to date, there is indirect evidence that at least the "core" questions on the PSP surveys solicit responses reliably (i.e., consistently).

The issue of the validity of the data from the PSP surveys is quite another matter. As indicated earlier, the data obtained from the PSP surveys are self-reports from participating physicians. This poses two questions of particular importance for this study: Do physicians really know the answers to the questions asked of them on the PSP surveys? Do they accurately report that information, or do they overreport some information (i.e., the number of hours they work per week), while they underreport other information (i.e., their net annual incomes)?

To some extent the latter issue was addressed by Nelson, Jacobs, and Breer (1975) when they compared the results of data collected on 13 primary care physicians for a one-week period. They used a task inventory to collect one set of data, a process in which the physicians under study self-reported at the end of the week the frequency and duration of the tasks which they had performed during the week. Their other data collection technique involved using trained observers to "shadow" the 13 primary care physicians and complete checklists and other time and motion study protocols on the physicians during the same week. The study reports a considerable disparity between the time allocations obtained from the two data collection techniques. Further, Nelson, Jacobs, and Breer (1975, 111) claim that the major reason for the disparity is "a tendency of some physicians to over-estimate both the frequency and duration of tasks relative to the observer." Accordingly, they question the validity of using the task inventory or self-report method when collecting data on physician practice patterns and suggest that other observational methods would be more valid.

The former issue (physicians' knowledge of the issue in question) is similar. That is, in addition to the problem of physicians overestimating the amount of time that they spend performing a variety of tasks, one may question whether these same physicians can provide valid data on other patient characteristics. One particular concern here has been physicians' estimates of the amount of time that patients have to wait to schedule an appointment to see the physician or the amount of time that patients must wait in the office upon arriving for the scheduled visit. Critics of the PSP survey data allege that physicians do not really know this information because the physician neither schedules the appointments nor observes when the patient first arrives at the office waiting room.

The results of several national surveys, however, suggest the opposite. Indeed, compare the physician estimates of patient queues taken from PSP–14 with patient estimates of patient queues taken from a 1981 Gallup public opinion survey and with physician estimates of patient queues taken from a 1981 Market Opinion Research (MOR) physician opinion survey. They demonstrate the validity of the PSP–14 data and our use of them in this study. The results of these comparisons are shown in table 2.2. These data clearly indicate the close correspondence between estimates of patient queues obtained from physicians in PSP–14 and those obtained from patients interviewed face-to-face in the Gallup Survey and from physicians interviewed by telephone in the MOR survey. Unfortunately, because the Gallup and MOR surveys do not collect detailed information on the physicians' practice settings, we cannot make more extensive comparisons. Similarly, although the physicians' estimates of patient queues obtained in PSP–14 closely approximate those reported by patients in the National Health Care Expenditure Study (NHCES 1981), we cannot make direct comparisons here because the NHCES fails to distinguish between established and new patients. Nonetheless, we believe that the general comparisons shown in table 2.2 rather convincingly demonstrate the validity of using physicians' estimates of their patients' scheduling and office queues, and we assume that their knowledge in other patient-related areas is equally valid.

A further note is in order at this point. First, recall that the purpose of this monograph is to assess the effect of the organization of medical practice on the practice of medicine. Second, note that what Nelson, Jacobs, and Breer (1975)

Table 2.2   Comparison of estimates of patient queue measures obtained
from three surveys using different methods and respondent
populations

Patient Queue Measures	Surveys		
	PSP–14* (1980) Mail Questionnaires to Physicians	Gallup† (1981) Personal Interviews of Patients	MOR‡ (1981) Telephone Interviews of Physicians
Appointment scheduling (number of days waited by established patients)	4.5	4.6	4.8
Office waits (number of minutes waited to see the physician)	19.7	19.3	20.7

*Goldfarb, D., ed., *Profile of Medical Practice, 1981.* Chicago: American Medical Association, 1981.
† Gallup Organization, Inc., *Public Attitudes Toward Health Care and Health Care Issues.* Princeton, NJ: Gallup, 1981.
‡ Market Opinion Research, Inc., *Physicians' Perceptions of Issues in Health Care and Medicine.* Detroit: Market Opinion Research, 1981.

have shown is that the point estimates (i.e., the means) obtained by using physicians' retrospective self-reports are probably overstated. As an aside, it seems reasonable to assume that this overstatement may have resulted from the physicians including in their actual patient contact estimates the amount of time that they spent reviewing charts, writing case histories, and attending grand rounds. These time-consuming activities would not have been included in the "shadow" estimates. Regardless of the reason for the overestimation, however, the fact is that the retrospective self-reporting method does not appear to generate valid point estimates.

While the validity of the point estimates themselves may be questioned (e.g., the amount of time spent with patients may be overestimated), Nelson, Jacobs, and Breer present no empirical evidence to suggest that this tendency to overestimate is more or less pronounced across the different organizational settings in which physicians may practice. That is, physicians in staff model HMOs are no more or no less likely to over- or underestimate the amount of time that they spend with their patients than are solo practitioners or physicians in fee-for-service group practices. Thus, the differences between the point estimates for various groupings of physicians based on the organizational structure of their medical practices should be reliable and meaningful. Therefore, our use of the PSP survey data for addressing differences in the practice of medicine as self-reported by physicians is, indeed, appropriate. Accordingly, in this monograph we report primarily on differences between the point estimates for physicians in the various organizational structures, not on the point estimates themselves.

The PSP-14 Surveys

The data used in this monograph are taken from two PSP surveys. The data on fee-for-service physicians (as well as the data on a small number of prepaid physicians) are taken from PSP–14M conducted during 1980 by the AMA Center for Health Services Research and Development, as shown in table 2.1. The PSP–14M questionnaire was mailed to a 5 percent, single-stage, proportionately stratified (on medical specialty categories) random sample of nonfederal, office-based physicians engaged in active medical practice in the United States. The sample was taken directly from the Masterfile's enumeration of every physician, regardless of AMA membership, in the United States. By using a series of four follow-up mailings at approximately monthly intervals, a usable completion rate of 50 percent was obtained, providing data on 5,133 physicians. Analytic comparisons of the medical specialty, census division, age, and sex of the responding physicians to the physician population have been shown to reveal no statistically significant differences (see Goldfarb 1981). Accordingly, the PSP–14M data provide an appropriate data source with which to empirically assess the impact of organizational structure on the practice of medicine.

Because only a few HMO physicians were likely to be included in PSP–14M, a special oversample of HMO physicians was designed. Obtaining comparable data from physicians practicing in HMOs involved two stages. First, a letter was sent to all HMOs listed in the *1978 Census of HMOs* compiled by the federal Office of Health Maintenance Organizations (OHMO 1978). The executive directors of each of the 203 HMOs enumerated in the *Census* were asked to provide a list of all physicians participating in their plans. Ninety-seven (48 percent) of the executive directors in the HMOs responded, and an additional 17 lists (8 percent) were obtained from the Registry of Group Practice study concurrently being conducted by the AMA. An analytic comparison of the response rates for the three major types of HMOs (i.e., the federal designations of staff models, group models, and IPAs) at this stage of the sampling process failed to indicate any nonresponse biases. That is, none of the three major types of HMOs were over- or under-represented with regard to the physician lists provided.

Second, a 20 percent sample was selected by systematically choosing one out of every five physicians from each of the 114 HMO physician lists, using a new random seed within each HMO. The HMO physician sample was then sent a standard PSP–14M questionnaire during 1980. Using four follow-up mailings to non-responding physicians at approximately monthly intervals, a usable response rate of 50 percent was obtained, resulting in a sample of 1,642 HMO physicians. Based on the then most current categorization published by the OHMO in the *Federal Register*, responding physicians were initially classified as participating in either group model, staff model, or IPA model HMOs. Subsequently, the group model HMO category was further disaggregated into Kaiser and non-Kaiser group model HMOs. On known criteria, which are admittedly few and not very specific (indeed at the time that these data were collected, HMO physician population parameters were essentially limited to the type of HMO and its census division), the resulting sample of HMO physicians (PSP–14H) was representative of the population of HMO physicians (see Wolinsky and Corry 1981). Thus, although unknown biases are possible, PSP–14H appears to be an appropriate data source with which to assess the impact of organizational structure on the practice of medicine.

Pooling the PSP–14M and PSP–14H physician surveys constitutes the data set used in this monograph, and it is hereafter referred to simply as PSP–14. In the pooled PSP–14 data set are 6,691 responding physicians; 196 may be identified as practicing in Kaiser model HMOs, 176 in non-Kaiser group model HMOs, 163 in staff model HMOs, 1,159 in independent practice associations or IPAs, 2,507 in solo fee-for-service, and 2,490 in group fee-for-service settings.

Basic Cross-tabular Results

Table 2.3 shows the number of respondents by medical specialty and organization of medical practice for the 6,691 physicians in the pooled PSP–14 data set. There are two important facts that should be gleaned from table 2.3. First, the distributions of physicians by medical specialty across the six organizational settings in which medicine is practiced are, for the most part, comparable. That is, the relative frequency of physicians in each of the nine specialties is about the same across each of the six practice settings. For example, about 21 percent of the Kaiser model HMO physicians are in internal medicine, compared with 28 percent of the non-Kaiser group model HMO physicians, 23 percent of the staff model HMO physicians, 22 percent of the IPA physicians, 18 percent of the solo fee-for-service physicians, and 18 percent of the group fee-for-service physicians. Similar results occur in comparing the percentage distributions of the other eight medical specialties across the six organizational practice settings.

The second point discovered in table 2.3 is that for the Kaiser model HMOs, the non-Kaiser group model HMOs, and the staff model HMOs, the numbers of physicians in the radiology, psychiatry, anesthesiology, and other medical specialty categories are insignificant for analytic purposes. That is, for the nonresidual medical specialties just listed, there are always fewer than ten physicians in the cells for these three HMO types. Accordingly, in the multivariate analysis that will be reported in chapters 3 and 4, radiologists, psychiatrists, anesthesiologists, and the residual category of other medical specialties will be excluded from the analysis to eliminate the problem of estimating effects across empty or nearly empty cells. For the remainder of the simple cross-tabular analyses presented in this chapter, however, these four medical specialty categories will be included because we will also be presenting the 95 percent confidence intervals around the point estimates, thus reflecting the instability associated with those point estimates. Thus, the tables subsequently presented in this chapter contain not only the point estimates but also the confidence intervals around those estimates, indicating the imprecision associated with calculating means based on such thinly populated sampling cells.

Table 2.4 presents the average total number of hours practiced per week by medical specialty and the organization of medical practice. These data indicate that the practice of medicine, at least as indicated by the total number of hours worked per week, does vary by both medical specialty and the practice setting. The effects of medical specialty can be seen by comparing the average number of hours *within a given column*, representing differences within a particular practice setting. For example, comparing the average number of hours down the column for Kaiser model HMO physicians indicates that internists spend about ten more hours per week on average than do their general or family practice counterparts. Other column-based comparisons also reveal differences, although the magnitudes are not as great. For example, the difference between the average number of hours worked per week by internists and general or family practitioners in solo fee-for-service practice settings is only about four hours, which appears to be the more common difference reflected in the four remaining practice settings as well.

Comparing the average number of hours practiced per week *within a given row* (i.e., within a particular medical specialty) indicates the effect of the practice setting on the practice of medicine. For example, comparing the average total number of hours across the six practice settings for general or family practice physicians indicates that Kaiser group model HMO physicians have the shortest average work weeks, with physicians in IPAs and in either form of fee-for-service practice having the longest average work weeks. Although the pattern does not hold for all medical specialties, two points warrant further attention. First, there are meaningful differences in the average total number of hours practiced per week by physicians in the same specialty in different practice settings. Thus, the data in table 2.4 demonstrate that when medical specialties are controlled, *there are differences based on the organization of medical practice* in terms of how many hours a physician works per week. Second, for the five medical specialties in which there are an adequate number of cases (general or family practice, internal medicine, surgery, pediatrics, and obstetrics/gynecology), the differences are usually such that the fee-for-service physicians work longer weeks than the HMO physicians. Fee-for-

Table 2.3   Number of respondents, by medical specialty and organization of medical practice

Medical Specialty	Kaiser Group Model HMOs	Non-Kaiser Group Model HMOs	Staff Model HMOs	Independent Practice Associations	Group Fee-for-Service	Solo Fee-for-Service	Total
General or family practice	18 (9%)	13 (7%)	19 (12%)	189 (16%)	371 (15%)	611 (24%)	1,221 (18%)
Internal medicine	41 (21)	49 (28)	37 (23)	260 (22)	445 (18)	462 (18)	1,294 (19)
Surgery	36 (18)	36 (20)	40 (25)	288 (25)	529 (21)	602 (24)	1,531 (23)
Pediatrics	27 (14)	28 (16)	19 (12)	120 (10)	210 (8)	112 (4)	516 (8)
Obstetrics/ gynecology	16 (8)	16 (9)	19 (12)	95 (8)	204 (8)	174 (7)	524 (8)
Radiology	8 (4)	4 (2)	4 (2)	54 (5)	181 (7)	31 (1)	282 (4)
Psychiatry	9 (5)	9 (5)	8 (5)	57 (5)	125 (5)	248 (10)	456 (7)
Anesthesiology	6 (3)	4 (2)	4 (2)	27 (2)	121 (5)	90 (4)	252 (4)
Other	35 (18)	17 (10)	13 (8)	69 (6)	304 (12)	177 (7)	615 (9)
Total	196 (100%)	176 (100%)	163 (100%)	1,159 (100%)	2,490 (100%)	2,507 (100%)	6,691 (100%)

Table 2.4 Total number of hours practiced per week, by medical specialty and organization of medical practice

Medical Specialty	Kaiser Group Model HMOs	Non-Kaiser Group Model HMOs	Staff Model HMOs	Independent Practice Associations	Group Fee-for-Service	Solo Fee-for-Service
General or family practice	38.5 ±4.0	44.2 ±5.7	43.5 ±3.3	48.1 ±1.6	49.9 ±1.3	47.0 ±1.3
Internal medicine	48.2 ±2.8	48.6 ±3.4	47.1 ±3.5	51.6 ±1.5	53.4 ±5.6	51.0 ±1.0
Surgery	46.8 ±5.6	51.6 ±4.1	53.5 ±4.3	52.8 ±1.5	54.5 ±1.2	49.6 ±1.2
Pediatrics	47.3 ±3.4	47.6 ±3.9	49.1 ±6.7	48.5 ±2.2	48.1 ±1.9	48.5 ±2.2
Obstetrics/ gynecology	47.3 ±5.3	47.7 ±7.5	54.7 ±5.9	53.5 ±2.9	52.6 ±2.2	47.6 ±2.8
Radiology	43.9 ±5.5	50.5 ±7.8	34.5 ±12.8	47.3 ±1.9	47.8 ±1.4	43.7 ±3.8
Psychiatry	44.2 ±6.6	45.2 ±3.1	43.4 ±4.1	50.3 ±4.1	44.9 ±2.2	45.8 ±1.6
Anesthesiology	45.7 ±7.8	50.0 ±6.4	49.7 ±15.6	51.6 ±3.7	52.0 ±1.8	48.8 ±2.7
Other	43.0 ±2.6	43.3 ±5.0	45.3 ±6.2	47.2 ±2.7	47.3 ±1.4	44.7 ±2.0

Note: Calculated in actual hours, with 95% confidence intervals shown.

service includes IPA physicians, because that is how they are generally reimbursed for their prepaid patients. Thus, these data suggest that there may be a pattern of relationships between the organization of medical practice and the practice of medicine.

To address this issue further, we shall present three more sets of tables that deal with physician incomes and expenses, patient queues, and the amount of time physicians spend with their patients. Tables 2.5 and 2.6 present the physicians' 1979 net income and gross expenses by their medical specialty and practice setting. The entries in tables 2.5 and 2.6 are expressed in thousands of dollars, with 95 percent confidence intervals shown. With regard to net income, table 2.5 shows that income (just like the number of hours in the average work week) is related to medical specialty even when we control for the organization of medical practice. Further, this relationship holds across all practice settings. For example, among the Kaiser model HMO physicians the two medical specialties with the highest 1979 net incomes are obstetrics/gynecology and surgery. Moreover, this pattern holds for all five of the other practice settings. Similarly, general or family practitioners and pediatricians have the lowest net incomes across the practice settings.

The second point that was observed for the length of the average work week (see table 2.4) also holds for income (see table 2.5). That is, comparing 1979 net incomes within a given row shows that there is considerable variation in how much physicians of the same medical specialty earn in different practice settings. Once again, it is generally true that physicians who are reimbursed on a fee-for-service basis have higher net incomes than those who work in prepaid health care delivery systems.

The data on professional expenses shown in table 2.6 are comparable, although the magnitude of the differences is, for the most part, far more striking. For example, among internists the average gross expenses reported among Kaiser model HMO physicians are about $2,400 compared with about $50,000 in the fee-for-service setting. Similarly, the professional expenses for general or family practitioners in prepaid health care delivery systems average less than $25,000 compared with an average of more than $60,000 in the fee-for-service settings. These data, however, are difficult to interpret because they probably reflect more on the fringe benefit package associated with prepaid health care delivery settings, where malpractice insurance and other professional expenses are more likely to be paid by the corporations rather than by the individual physicians. However, if this were indeed the case we would anticipate that the average gross expenses for physicians practicing in group fee-for-service settings would be less than for their counterparts in solo fee-for-service settings or in IPAs. This, however, is not the case. (We shall return to this issue in chapter 4 with a more elaborate multivariate analysis.)

Tables 2.7 through 2.9 present data on three aspects of patient queues by medical specialty and the practice setting in which the physician works. In par-

Table 2.5 1979 net income, by medical specialty and organization of medical practice

Medical Specialty	Kaiser Group Model HMOs	Non-Kaiser Group Model HMOs	Staff Model HMOs	Independent Practice Associations	Group Fee-for-Service	Solo Fee-for-Service
General or family practice	57.3 ± 7.5	49.7 ± 6.0	42.3 ± 8.4	62.8 ± 4.8	61.6 ± 2.9	61.9 ± 3.7
Internal medicine	70.7 ± 6.5	57.5 ± 5.8	60.8 ± 7.4	76.2 ± 4.6	77.4 ± 4.5	74.5 ± 4.4
Surgery	74.4 ± 7.7	88.0 ± 16.7	82.1 ± 15.0	97.7 ± 6.6	101.5 ± 4.5	90.0 ± 4.7
Pediatrics	68.1 ± 10.2	53.6 ± 8.4	54.9 ± 9.2	60.0 ± 4.5	60.1 ± 3.5	58.8 ± 5.9
Obstetrics/ gynecology	81.0 ± 14.3	73.5 ± 13.3	66.8 ± 15.7	96.1 ± 9.7	92.4 ± 6.4	87.8 ± 9.7
Radiology	69.3 ± 15.1	69.0 ± 17.8	64.5 ± 29.1	97.4 ± 9.3	98.0 ± 12.4	97.2 ± 21.7
Psychiatry	63.6 ± 12.3	50.0 ± 8.1	51.3 ± 9.8	66.1 ± 11.3	57.3 ± 4.8	65.3 ± 5.5
Anesthesiology	84.5 ± 23.5	73.8 ± 13.5	77.8 ± 23.2	98.9 ± 13.7	87.8 ± 6.0	96.4 ± 9.1
Other	72.8 ± 7.7	62.2 ± 12.3	64.1 ± 15.2	78.4 ± 8.4	74.5 ± 4.2	73.6 ± 7.4

Note: Calculated in thousands of dollars, with 95% confidence intervals shown.

Table 2.6 1979 gross expenses, by medical specialty and organization of medical practice

Medical Specialty	Kaiser Group Model HMOs	Non-Kaiser Group Model HMOs	Staff Model HMOs	Independent Practice Associations	Group Fee-for-Service	Solo Fee-for-Service
General or family practice	23.6 ± 43.2	10.6 ± 19.3	22.3 ± 19.2	70.0 ± 8.3	65.6 ± 8.8	50.3 ± 4.2
Internal medicine	2.4 ± 1.1	47.0 ± 39.1	33.1 ± 13.3	57.7 ± 7.6	55.5 ± 8.4	51.1 ± 4.1
Surgery	3.8 ± 2.9	71.0 ± 27.2	71.6 ± 29.2	65.9 ± 8.1	76.8 ± 8.2	63.2 ± 4.6
Pediatrics	3.5 ± 2.6	28.7 ± 29.0	30.7 ± 35.0	42.8 ± 6.1	51.0 ± 10.6	51.0 ± 6.2
Obstetrics/gynecology	38.3 ± 73.0	31.2 ± 29.7	23.3 ± 15.9	78.9 ± 13.5	72.4 ± 15.7	60.0 ± 8.3
Radiology	1.7 ± 3.3	150.5 ± 293.0	92.7 ± 114.1	45.3 ± 25.5	47.8 ± 15.9	39.6 ± 19.2
Psychiatry	10.3 ± 13.6	6.7 ± 6.7	11.3 ± 7.5	24.8 ± 8.4	30.1 ± 14.5	20.5 ± 2.1
Anesthesiology	1.3 ± 0.5	—	21.3 ± 18.4	32.3 ± 9.2	23.0 ± 7.5	29.8 ± 6.6
Other	5.0 ± 4.8	10.3 ± 9.2	29.0 ± 21.8	54.2 ± 20.9	25.2 ± 7.0	51.4 ± 10.7

Note: Calculated in thousands of dollars, with 95% confidence intervals shown.

ticular, tables 2.7 and 2.8 present data on the actual number of days that new and established patients, respectively, have to wait for a scheduled appointment with their physician. These tables yield three interesting comparisons. The first two are similar to those that we have made in the previous tables. That is, comparison of entries in the cells within rows of the data shows that across different practice settings, physicians of the same medical specialty have different patient queues, on average. For example, in solo fee-for-service settings new patients have to wait about 3 days and established patients about 2 days to see their general or family practitioners; in Kaiser model HMOs the wait is nearly 12 days for new patients and almost 7 days for established patients. Similarly, the patient queues depicted in tables 2.7 and 2.8 within columns vary considerably depending upon the medical specialty of the physician. For example, the patient queues for new and established patients are shortest for general and family practitioners, and longest for patients waiting to see an obstetrician/gynecologist.

The third comparison that can be made between tables 2.7 and 2.8 reveals the differences in patient queues facing new as opposed to established patients. To demonstrate this, one need only compare the new patient queues shown in table 2.7 for a general or family physician in a Kaiser model HMO with the established patient queues shown in table 2.8 for the same type of practitioner in the same practice setting. In this example, new patients have to wait about 12 days compared with 7 days for established patients. This preferential treatment for established patients holds for all medical specialties and for all practice settings.

The data presented in table 2.9 demonstrate, by their contrast with the data in tables 2.7 and 2.8, the fact that waiting room queues are a different phenomenon than scheduling queues. That is, while scheduling queues clearly vary by medical specialty and the organization of medical practice, waiting room queues are far more homogeneous across medical specialties and practice settings. There is some variation in the waiting room queues for general or family practitioners across the six practice settings, but that variation is not large. Similarly, while there is some variation in the waiting room queues across medical specialties within the same practice settings, that variation is also not large. This suggests that waiting room queues result from either a stochastic or unpredictable set of factors or a uniform set of factors unrelated to medical specialty or practice settings. This is in stark contrast to scheduling queues, which are clearly related to and predictable by medical specialty and the organization of medical practice.

The average number of minutes that physicians spend per patient in the office and in the hospital also varies by medical specialty and practice setting, as shown in tables 2.10 and 2.11. For example, for the most part solo fee-for-service physicians spend more time with their patients regardless of their medical specialty than physicians in the other practice settings, especially when we look at office visits (table 2.10), but also when we look at hospital visits (table 2.11).

Table 2.7 New patient waiting time to schedule an appointment, by medical specialty and organization of medical practice

Medical Specialty	Kaiser Group Model HMOs	Non-Kaiser Group Model HMOs	Staff Model HMOs	Independent Practice Associations	Group Fee-for-Service	Solo Fee-for-Service
General or family practice	11.7 ±6.7	6.5 ±3.9	9.3 ±4.1	4.4 ±0.8	4.6 ±0.8	3.1 ±0.6
Internal medicine	34.0 ±8.2	19.0 ±6.4	8.5 ±2.8	8.1 ±1.4	13.2 ±2.6	8.0 ±1.4
Surgery	22.2 ±7.4	11.9 ±4.5	14.5 ±7.8	7.2 ±1.3	9.7 ±1.5	7.5 ±1.3
Pediatrics	23.2 ±8.1	9.8 ±5.7	12.4 ±5.7	8.5 ±2.6	7.8 ±1.5	5.3 ±2.0
Obstetrics/gynecology	52.2 ±31.9	31.5 ±13.9	20.5 ±7.8	14.0 ±2.9	15.6 ±2.5	9.5 ±2.6
Radiology	18.0 ±11.8	4.7 ±4.6	2.0 ±1.9	2.5 ±3.3	1.2 ±0.5	1.7 ±1.5
Psychiatry	23.8 ±9.1	17.1 ±13.7	6.9 ±7.8	10.6 ±4.0	8.2 ±1.3	8.9 ±3.4
Anesthesiology	0.5 ±1.0	–	–	0.9 ±1.0	5.6 ±9.5	0.9 ±1.0
Other	21.5 ±9.5	13.3 ±13.0	14.9 ±12.0	6.8 ±1.9	6.7 ±1.9	5.3 ±2.0

Note: Calculated in actual number of days, with 95% confidence intervals shown.

Table 2.8 Established patient waiting time to schedule an appointment, by medical specialty and organization of medical practice

Medical Specialty	Kaiser Group Model HMOs	Non-Kaiser Group Model HMOs	Staff Model HMOs	Independent Practice Associations	Group Fee-for-Service	Solo Fee-for-Service
General or family practice	6.5±4.9	3.8±2.5	5.3±1.9	2.6±0.6	2.5±0.4	1.7±0.3
Internal medicine	16.4±5.6	10.7±4.0	5.6±2.4	3.6±0.7	4.6±0.9	2.8±0.5
Surgery	12.2±4.9	4.7±2.0	4.8±1.7	5.1±1.2	6.6±1.4	4.7±0.6
Pediatrics	17.3±7.6	6.5±4.2	6.7±3.2	5.3±2.1	5.1±1.3	3.3±1.8
Obstetrics/gynecology	32.3±11.8	22.0±11.7	7.6±3.0	12.6±3.7	13.7±2.5	6.7±1.6
Radiology	11.0±2.0	4.7±4.6	—	2.5±3.3	0.7±0.3	0.7±0.5
Psychiatry	7.1±3.2	4.9±3.5	3.7±2.6	5.3±2.9	4.0±1.0	2.7±0.4
Anesthesiology	0.5±1.0	—	—	0.9±1.0	0.7±0.8	1.0±1.0
Other	8.9±4.5	7.9±6.4	6.9±4.8	3.3±1.3	3.9±1.5	2.7±0.6

Note: Calculated in actual number of days, with 95% confidence intervals shown.

Table 2.9   Patient waiting time after arrival, by medical specialty and organization of medical practice

Medical Specialty	Kaiser Group Model HMOs	Non-Kaiser Group Model HMOs	Staff Model HMOs	Independent Practice Associations	Group Fee-for-Service	Solo Fee-for-Service
General or family practice	20.8 ± 7.8	16.2 ± 3.3	20.7 ± 5.1	21.1 ± 1.8	25.2 ± 1.7	22.8 ± 1.3
Internal medicine	15.0 ± 3.3	17.2 ± 5.0	18.7 ± 4.5	19.8 ± 2.2	20.6 ± 1.5	17.7 ± 1.3
Surgery	15.2 ± 3.0	16.6 ± 3.2	19.7 ± 3.7	20.2 ± 1.5	24.2 ± 1.4	19.8 ± 1.2
Pediatrics	13.7 ± 3.1	16.2 ± 4.6	17.8 ± 6.6	19.1 ± 2.3	22.3 ± 2.0	20.4 ± 2.3
Obstetrics/ gynecology	17.8 ± 4.4	18.9 ± 4.8	20.5 ± 4.7	23.6 ± 2.6	24.7 ± 1.8	20.3 ± 1.7
Radiology	15.0 ± 0.0	21.7 ± 8.6	5.0 ± 0.0	14.7 ± 3.3	18.7 ± 2.3	16.7 ± 5.2
Psychiatry	2.7 ± 2.8	16.3 ± 14.3	2.9 ± 3.6	4.77 ± 1.7	8.0 ± 2.1	4.3 ± 0.9
Anesthesiology	26.0 ± 43.4	—	—	4.29 ± 5.4	12.2 ± 6.0	4.9 ± 4.1
Other	15.5 ± 4.0	12.4 ± 9.0	12.6 ± 1.9	18.0 ± 4.0	17.6 ± 2.5	17.5 ± 1.8

Note: Calculated in actual number of minutes, with 95% confidence intervals shown.

Similarly, when we compare the average amount of time spent per patient within a column (i.e., controlling for practice setting and looking at the effects of medical specialty), we find that internists and surgeons consistently spend more time per patient in the office, while surgeons and obstetrician/gynecologists spend more time per patient in the hospital. Thus, the data in tables 2.10 and 2.11 provide additional evidence for the relationship between the organization of medical practice and the practice of medicine, controlling for the effects of medical specialty.

Table 2.12 presents data that bear more directly on the potential issue of why physicians choose one practice setting over another. In PSP–14 the physicians were asked to indicate how important several issues were to their choice of solo or group practice. The issues listed were: (1) the business side of medical practice, (2) the predictability of a practice schedule, (3) personal autonomy in delivering care, (4) practice location, and (5) earnings potential. Following Wolinsky (1982), these questions may be used as proxies for self-selection.

The data in table 2.12 demonstrate that the self-selection issue is an important one that must be addressed in examining the effect of the organization of medical practice on the practice of medicine. As indicated in table 2.12, there are clear differences in the attitudinal characteristics of physicians in the six different practice settings. In particular, on the business, predictability, and autonomy issues there is a nearly perfect monotonic relationship between the importance of the issues and the position of the practice setting on the bureaucratic-autonomous dimension. The business and predictability issues are positively related, and the personal autonomy issue is negatively related to this underlying dimension. The data on the importance of practice location and earnings potential, however, are mixed, suggesting that these issues are not important discriminators in physicians' choices of practice settings.

Summary and Discussion

There were two important points to be made in this chapter. The first was to identify the data to be used in this study, describe the technique used to obtain them, and discuss their reliability and validity for our subsequent analyses. The second was to present some basic cross-tabular analyses of various aspects of these data in order to demonstrate in an intuitive fashion that there are differences in the practice of medicine depending upon the organizational setting in which physicians work, even after adjusting for differences in medical specialty.

We have not discussed each of the cross-tabular presentations in great detail because they represent an oversimplification of the realities associated with the effects of the organization of medical practice on the practice of medicine. Just as it is necessary to control for the effect of medical specialty when examining differences in the practice of medicine across the six practice settings, it is necessary

Table 2.10 Time spent per patient in the office, by medical specialty and organization of medical practice

Medical Specialty	Kaiser Group Model HMOs	Non-Kaiser Group Model HMOs	Staff Model HMOs	Independent Practice Associations	Group Fee-for-Service	Solo Fee-for-Service
General or family practice	18.8 ± 1.9	20.5 ± 2.8	22.6 ± 3.4	23.1 ± 2.6	20.5 ± 1.2	22.9 ± 1.2
Internal medicine	24.2 ± 1.8	27.2 ± 4.7	26.4 ± 4.1	30.5 ± 2.3	32.9 ± 3.3	32.6 ± 2.1
Surgery	26.5 ± 5.5	24.5 ± 5.4	27.1 ± 4.7	24.6 ± 1.8	21.5 ± 1.1	28.4 ± 3.8
Pediatrics	20.5 ± 2.1	19.2 ± 2.0	25.5 ± 6.3	23.1 ± 3.6	25.9 ± 5.5	19.5 ± 1.9
Obstetrics/ gynecology	16.7 ± 1.9	20.0 ± 3.2	26.5 ± 4.7	20.2 ± 2.2	19.9 ± 1.6	25.1 ± 2.4
Radiology	75.2 ± 91.6	—	18.9 ± 3.9	16.0 ± 8.7	17.2 ± 3.7	31.1 ± 22.2
Psychiatry	64.5 ± 7.2	59.5 ± 17.7	55.3 ± 11.1	60.8 ± 7.8	60.4 ± 7.1	62.5 ± 6.8
Anesthesiology	—	—	—	57.0 ± 64.7	37.2 ± 24.2	51.6 ± 53.3
Other	27.8 ± 10.2	36.1 ± 16.0	33.9 ± 10.3	27.6 ± 7.0	32.4 ± 4.8	31.0 ± 4.7

Note: Calculated in actual number of minutes, with 95% confidence intervals shown.

Table 2.11 Time spent per patient visit in the hospital, by medical specialty and organization of medical practice

Medical Specialty	Kaiser Group Model HMOs	Non-Kaiser Group Model HMOs	Staff Model HMOs	Independent Practice Associations	Group Fee-for-Service	Solo Fee-for-Service
General or family practice	57.4±47.6	62.3±24.5	65.2±29.8	44.5±7.5	37.2±5.6	47.4±5.7
Internal medicine	34.5±8.8	43.6±12.3	60.6±22.5	38.2±3.6	38.0±3.8	43.2±4.3
Surgery	54.4±15.3	56.1±13.6	70.0±17.6	57.6±6.2	58.6±5.4	67.2±10.2
Pediatrics	40.3±13.3	60.2±24.5	47.2±14.7	44.7±8.3	46.6±8.8	64.1±12.6
Obstetrics/gynecology	52.6±21.3	43.6±14.5	80.5±24.4	56.3±8.3	57.1±7.5	73.1±12.7
Radiology	—	—	—	21.6±13.1	25.8±8.4	29.2±19.3
Psychiatry	69.0±25.6	44.0±13.3	90.2±73.7	55.9±16.2	48.9±5.3	59.9±8.7
Anesthesiology	88.4±75.3	87.7±122.1	79.3±72.9	66.3±19.4	63.2±11.6	78.9±14.3
Other	31.8±12.4	51.8±56.4	46.9±18.9	83.8±37.1	42.1±9.6	53.4±9.0

Note: Calculated in actual number of minutes, with 95% confidence intervals shown.

Table 2.12 Percent of physicians who rate various issues as "very important" in their choice of a practice setting, by practice setting

Medical Specialty	Kaiser Group Model HMOs	Non-Kaiser Group Model HMOs	Staff Model HMOs	Independent Practice Associations	Group Fee-for-Service	Solo Fee-for-Service
1. Business side of medical practice	34	31	29	28	28	22
2. Predictability of practice schedule	56	39	43	31	38	31
3. Personal autonomy in delivering care	28	35	44	55	44	76
4. Practice location	49	44	44	35	38	40
5. Earnings potential	17	14	9	15	18	20

to control for additional factors, such as the age, sex, and geographic location of the physician, as well as for the self-selection issue. To do that simultaneously in a cross-tabular fashion, however, is difficult. In the next two chapters we rely on reasonably sophisticated multivariate techniques that allow us to partition out the effects of these other factors as well as those of medical specialty, so that we may estimate the net effects of the organization of medical practice on the practice of medicine. The purpose of these cross-tabular analyses, then, has been to demonstrate clearly what scholars know: *medical practice varies across practice settings.* In the remainder of this monograph, we concentrate on estimating precisely how much medical practice varies in different settings.

References

Carmines, Edward, and Richard Zeller. 1979. *Reliability and Validity Assessment.* Beverly Hills: Sage.

Gallup Organization. 1981. *Public Attitudes Toward Health Care and Health Care Issues.* Princeton, N.J.: Gallup.

Glandon, Gerald, and Roberta Shapiro. 1980a. "Relative changes in medical care prices: the Consumer Price Index, 1970–1979." In *Profile of Medical Practice, 1980,* edited by Gerald Glandon and Roberta Shapiro. Chicago: American Medical Association.

———. 1980b. "Trends in physicians' incomes, expenses, and fees: 1970–1979." In *Profile of Medical Practice, 1980,* edited by Gerald Glandon and Roberta Shapiro. Chicago: American Medical Association.

———. 1980c. *Profile of Medical Practice, 1980.* Chicago: American Medical Association.

Glandon, Gerald, and Jack Werner. 1980. "Physicians' practice experience during the decade of the 1970s." *Journal of the American Medical Association* 244:2514–18.

Goldfarb, David, ed. 1981. *Profile of Medical Practice, 1981.* Chicago: American Medical Association.

Goodman, Louis, and Barry Eisenberg. 1977. "The quality of physician data." *Review of Public Data Use* 5:37–44.

Goodman, Louis, and Lynn Jensen. 1981. "The American Medical Association's Periodic Survey of Physicians." In *Profile of Medical Practice, 1981,* edited by David Goldfarb. Chicago: American Medical Association.

Jensen, Lynn; Lorna Wunderman; and Louis Goodman. 1982. *Characteristics of Physicians, December 31, 1979.* 51 Volumes. (HRA 79–101 through HRA 79–151) Washington, D.C.: Government Printing Office.

Market Opinion Research, Inc. 1981. *Physicians' Perceptions of Issues of Health Care and Medicine.* Detroit: Market Opinion Research.

National Health Care Examination Survey (NHCES). 1981. *Waiting Times in Different Medical Settings: Appointment Waits and Office Waits.* Data Preview 6. Washington, D.C.: National Center for Health Services Research.

Nelson, Eugene; Arthur Jacobs; and Paul Breer. 1975. "A study of the validity of the task inventory method of job analysis." *Medical Care* 13:104–13.

Office of Health Maintenance Organizations (OHMO). 1978. *Census of Prepaid Plans, 1978.* Washington, D.C.: Government Printing Office.

Theodore, Chris, and G. Sutter. 1966. "A report on the first Periodic Survey of Physicians." *Journal of the American Medical Association* 202:516–24.

Wolinsky, Fredric. 1982. "Why physicians choose different types of practice settings." *Health Services Research* 17:399–419.

Wolinsky, Fredric, and Barbara Corry. 1981. "Organizational structure and medical practice in health maintenance organizations." In *Profile of Medical Practice, 1981*, edited by David Goldfarb. Chicago: American Medical Association.

3

The Organization of Medical Practice, Patient Queues, and Time Spent with Patients

Overview

The purpose of this chapter is threefold. First, we describe the data and the specifications of the regression equations used in operationalizing the general analytic model to assess the effects of the organization of medical practice on patient queues and time spent with patients. Second, we use the general analytic model to focus on the effects of the organization of medical practice on patient queues. In particular, we examine three aspects of patient queues: (1) the amount of time it takes for new patients to schedule routine office visits, (2) the amount of time it takes for established patients to schedule routine office visits, and (3) the amount of time patients have to wait upon arrival at the physician's office for their scheduled appointments. Finally, we use the general analytic model to study the effects of the organization of medical practice on the amount of time that physicians spend with their patients. In particular, we separately examine average office and hospital visit lengths.

Operationalizing the Analytic Model for Patient Queues and Time Spent with Patients

As indicated in chapter 1, the general analytic model that guides this research is shown in its functional form in equation 1:

$$POM = f\ (SD,\ EN,\ AT,\ PS) \tag{1}$$

where *POM* refers to the practice of medicine, f denotes that the practice of medicine is a function of the characteristics shown in the following parenthetical statement, *SD* represents the sociodemographic characteristics of the physician, *EN* represents the environmental characteristics that may constrain a physician's opportunity to practice medicine, *AT* represents the attitudinal characteristics indicative of the physician's preference structure (reflecting upon the self-selection issues), and *PS* represents the practice setting in which the physician works (solo fee-for-service, group fee-for-service, IPA model HMOs, staff model HMOs, non-Kaiser group model HMOs, or Kaiser model HMOs). As discussed in chapter 2, the data used to empirically assess the general analytic model described in equation 1 are taken from the PSP–14 survey conducted by the Center for Health Services Research and Development of the American Medical Association (AMA) during 1980. The PSP-14 data contain detailed information on the sociodemographic, environmental, attitudinal, and practice setting characteristics of 6,691 physicians in the six practice settings described above. As indicated in chapter 2, however, there is an insufficient number of radiologists, phychiatrists, anesthesiologists, and other (i.e., residual) medical specialty categories for detailed statistical analyses. Accordingly, in assessing the general analytic model, physicians from these four medical specialties are excluded from the analysis. This reduces the working sample to 5,086 physicians.

For two very different reasons, the 1,531 surgeons are also excluded from further analyses. The first reason is the remarkable heterogeneity within this medical specialty, especially as it is classified in the PSP–14 data. In particular, the PSP-14 data make no distinction between general surgeons, specialty surgeons, and subspecialty surgeons. Thus, the "surgery" specialty in the PSP–14 data includes a wide range of physicians, from "general" surgeons, to pediatric cardiovascular surgeons, to opthalmological surgeons. The second reason is that they are distinctly different from any of the four remaining medical specialties. That is, general or family practitioners, internists, pediatricians, and obstetrician/gynecologists are typically referred to as primary care physicians; surgeons are not. Thus, excluding surgeons from the remainder of the analyses allows us to focus on primary care physicians, who are the backbone of most HMOs and other collaborative practices (see Freidson 1970; Wolinsky 1980; Wolinsky and Marder 1982a, 1982b, 1983a, 1983b). Accordingly, the remainder of our analyses treat the effects of the organization of medical practice on the practice of medicine by 3,555 primary care physicians, who are likely to be the principal physician providers in their health care settings.

Table 3.1 contains the means, standard deviations, and coding algorithms of the variables used to operationalize the general analytic model with respect to patient queues and time spent with patients. There are seven measures of the sociodemographic (*SD*) characteristics: sex, AMA membership, board certification, experience, and a set of three dummy variables to measure medical specialty. Sex is included as a dummy variable to control for the previously documented effects of being female on physician work patterns (see Kehrer 1976; Langwell

1982; Wolinsky and Marder 1983b). About 6 percent of the primary care physicians in our sample are female. AMA membership and board certification are included as dummy variables in order to adjust for differences between individual and group conflict resolution preferences, as well as for a willingness to voluntarily submit to peer review mechanisms. That is, following Freshnock and Goodman (1980), we assume that membership in the AMA indicates more of a group orientation to the resolution of issues facing American medicine, and that board certification demonstrates a willingness on the part of the physician to be peer-reviewed. About 62 percent of the physicians in our sample are members of the AMA, and about 61 percent are board certified.

Experience is included in the general analytic model as the number of years that have passed since the physician completed the medical degree (M.D.). It has been shown (see Hall 1946, 1949) that physician practice patterns change as physicians progress through the various stages in the life and career cycle. The physicians in our sample had an average of 22.7 years of experience. To control for case-mix variations, even though the analysis has been restricted to primary care physicians, we include a set of dummy variables for internal medicine, pediatrics, and obstetrics/gynecology (which comprise 36 percent, 15 percent, and 15 percent of our sample, respectively). The medical specialty category omitted, in order to preserve the singularity of the correlation matrix, is general or family practice (which comprises 34 percent of our sample). Thus, the regression coefficients for each of these dummy variables indicate the difference between being in that particular medical specialty and being in general or family practice.

There are four measures of the environmental characteristics shown in table 3.1. The first is a dummy variable that we use to control for geographic variations in medical practice. Luft (1981, 1983; see also Wolinsky 1982) has shown that HMOs in particular, and group practices in general, are found more often in the western United States than anywhere else. Accordingly, the western United States variable adjusts the data for the greater affinity of the Pacific census region for HMOs and group practices. About 27 percent of the physicians in our sample are practicing in the Pacific census region. The second measure of the environmental characteristics is the physician-to-population ratio. This measure is calculated as the ratio of the number of physicians in the county during 1970 to the 1970 county population (in hundreds). The physician-to-population ratio allows us to adjust the data for the availability of medical care (i.e., for the level of competition among physicians for patients in their particular community setting). The average physician-to-population ratio in our sample was approximately .24, or about one physician for every 417 people in the county.

The third measure of the environmental characteristics is the 1975 average per capita income (in thousands of dollars) in the county. This measure allows us to adjust for differences in the demand for medical care services because it

Table 3.1   Means, standard deviations, and coding algorithms of the variables in the general analytic model (N=3,555)

Variables	Mean	Standard Deviation	Coding Algorithm
Sociodemographic characteristics (SD)			
Sex	.057	.232	1 = female 0 = male
AMA membership	.619	.486	1 = yes 0 = no
Board certified	.612	.487	1 = yes 0 = no
Experience	22.705	12.078	Actual number of years since receiving the M.D.
Internal medicine	.364	.481	1 = yes 0 = no
Pediatrics	.145	.352	1 = yes 0 = no
Obstetrics/Gynecology	.147	.355	1 = yes 0 = no
Environmental characteristics (EN)			
Western U.S.	.267	.442	1 = Pacific census region 0 = other census region
MD/POP ratio	.240	.165	Ratio of physicians in county to 1970 county population (in hundreds)
Local income	5.116	1.130	1975 average per capita income in county (in thousands)
Local education	11.975	.773	1970 median education in county (in years)
Attitudinal characteristics (AT)			
Business side of practice	.254	.435	1 = very important 0 = important or not important
Scheduling ease	.332	.471	1 = very important 0 = important or not important
Personal autonomy	.547	.498	1 = very important 0 = important or not important
Practice location	.367	.482	1 = very important 0 = important or not important
Earnings potential	.161	.367	1 = very important 0 = important or not important
Practice setting characteristics (PS)			
Kaiser model HMO	.029	.167	1 = yes 0 = no
Non-Kaiser group model HMO	.030	.170	1 = yes 0 = no

Table 3.1   Continued

Variables	Mean	Standard Deviation	Coding Algorithm
Staff model HMO	.026	.160	1 =yes 0 =no
IPA model HMO	.187	.390	1 =yes 0 =no
Solo F-F-S practice	.458	.498	1 =yes 0 =no
Patient queues			
Scheduling for routine office visits: new patients	8.934	16.878	Actual number of days (natural logarithms are used in the regression equations)
Scheduling for routine office visits: established patients	4.960	10.210	Actual number of days (natural logarithms are used in the regression equations)
Waiting time on arrival for scheduled appointments	21.110	14.914	Actual number of minutes (natural logarithms are used in the regression equations)
Length of physician visits			
In the office	25.656	21.316	Average number of minutes per patient (natural logarithms are used in the regression equations)
In the hospital	46.530	52.441	Average number of minutes per patient (natural logarithms are used in the regression equations)

allows us to hold average patient income levels constant. Average 1975 per capita income was $5,116. The fourth measure of the environmental characteristics is the 1970 median educational level (in years of schooling) in the county. This measure adjusts the data further for differences in patient pools by holding average patient educational levels constant. The median 1970 educational level was about 12 years of formal schooling. In addition to facilitating patient pool adjustments, the county income and education measures permit us, to some extent, to incorporate the sociodemographic characteristics of the patients into the general analytic model. That is, although the county income and educational level data are not specific to the patients of each particular physician, they do provide proxies of the patient pool available for each physician.

As shown in table 3.1, there are five measures of the attitudinal characteristics (or the self-selection issues). Physicians in our sample were asked to indicate how important each of these five issues were in their choice of solo versus group practice: were these issues very important, important, or not important? We then collapsed the responses into the dichotomy: very important versus important or not important. Of the physicians in our sample, 25.4 percent felt that the business side of practice was very important, 33.2 percent felt that scheduling ease was very important, 54.7 percent felt that personal autonomy was very important, 36.7 percent felt that practice location was very important, and 16.1 percent felt that earnings potential was very important in the selection of a practice setting. We use these five dichotomous measures to adjust the data for the self-selection issues. That is, these five measures allow us to control for differences in physicians' attitudinal compositions that may have led them to select certain practice settings over other practice settings. While they are not ideal measures of the self-selection issues (we would prefer to have measures of these variables at the time the decision was made), these five attitudinal items may reasonably be used as proxies.

The principal variables of interest in this study are the practice setting characteristics. They are measured by a set of five dummy variables reflecting the organizational settings in which the physicians practice medicine, including Kaiser model HMOs, non-Kaiser group model HMOs, staff model HMOs, IPA model HMOs, and solo fee-for-service practices. The omitted category in these regression analyses is the fee-for-service group practice. Thus, the regression coefficients for each of these five dummy variables indicate the difference of being in that particular practice setting rather than in fee-for-service group practice. In our sample, Kaiser model HMOs, non-Kaiser group model HMOs, and staff model HMOs each had about 3 percent of the total number of physicians. About 19 percent of the physicians were in IPA model HMOs, and about 46 percent were in solo fee-for-service practice settings. The remaining 27 percent of our sample were in fee-for-service group practices.

In this chapter our subject is the effect of the organization of medical practice on patient queues and the length of physician visits. The three measures of patient queues are: (1) the actual number of days it takes for new patients to schedule a routine office visit (about 8.9 days in our sample), (2) the actual number of days it takes for an established patient to schedule a routine office visit (about 5.0 days in our sample), and (3) the actual number of minutes that the patient has to wait on arrival in the office for the scheduled appointment (about 21.1 minutes in our sample). These data were obtained by asking the physicians in the PSP–14 surveys to report the average waiting times of their patients. Following an extensive analysis of the data, these three waiting-time measures were then transformed by taking their natural logarithms, which are more closely related to the independent variables than the original scalar values. Accordingly, although the means and standard deviations of the actual number of days (and minutes) are reported in table 3.1, the natural logarithms of these values are used in the subsequent regression analyses.

Also shown in table 3.1 are the two measures of the length of physician visits with their patients, both in the office and in the hospital. These variables were calculated from information contained on the PSP–14 questionnaires concerning the total number of hours worked in the office, the total number of patients seen in the office, the total number of hours worked in the hospital, and the total number of patients seen in the hospital. In both cases, physicians were asked to indicate the total number of hours (or visits) in their most recent complete week of practice. Overall, the average length of physician visits in the office was about 26 minutes, and the average length of physician visits in the hospital was about 47 minutes. Following an extensive analysis of the data, these two measures of the amount of time spent with patients were transformed by taking their natural logarithms, which are more closely related to the independent variables than the original scalar values. Although the average actual numbers of minutes per patient are reported in table 3.1, the natural logarithms of these numbers are used in the subsequent regression equations.

The Organization of Medical Practice and Patient Queues

To assess the effects of the general analytic model specified in equation 1 on patient queues, a set of three regression equations are used. In the first equation, hereafter referred to as model 1, the sociodemographic and environmental characteristics (*SD* and *EN*) are entered into the equation to predict patient queues. In the second equation, model 2, the attitudinal characteristics (*AT*) are added into the equation. In the third equation, model 3, the practice setting characteristics (*PS*) are added.

There are two particular advantages of using this hierarchical modeling strategy in assessing the effects of the organization of medical practice on patient queues, as well as the other medical practice characteristics for which the same approach will be used. (For a more detailed yet accessible discussion of these technical issues, see Lewis-Beck 1981.) First, the hierarchical modeling procedure permits the specific identification of the net contributions of the attitudinal (or self-selection) issues that go beyond the effects of the sociodemographic and environmental characteristics, as well as the net contributions of the practice setting characteristics that go beyond not only the sociodemographic and environmental characteristics, but beyond the attitudinal (or self-selection) issues as well. Subtracting the explained variance (i.e., R^2) obtained from model 1 from that obtained from model 2 indicates the net explanatory contribution made by the attitudinal characteristics. Similarly, subtracting the explained variance (R^2) obtained from model 2 from that obtained from model 3 indicates the net explanatory contribution of the practice setting characteristics. Thus, after subtracting the R^2 of model 2 from the R^2 of model 3, the remainder is truly the net effect on the practice of medicine associated specifically with the organization of medical practice.

Second, the hierarchical modeling approach helps assess whether the nature (the attitudinal characteristics) and the nurture (the practice setting characteristics) effects alter the original effects of the sociodemographic and environmental characteristics obtained from model 1. That is, did these effects (those of the *SD* and the *EN*) change when the attitudinal and practice setting characteristics were introduced? Similarly, this approach helps examine whether entering the practice setting characteristics in model 3 alters the effects obtained for the attitudinal characteristics from model 2. Thus, this hierarchical modeling approach permits us to assess the net contribution to the explained variance attributable to the attitudinal and practice setting characteristics. It also permits us to assess the extent to which the effects of the sociodemographic, environmental, and attitudinal characteristics may have been spurious, overestimated, or suppressed in the absence of the practice setting characteristics. For example, if the set of dummy variables for a medical specialty have a significant impact on the practice of medicine in model 1, but that significant impact is eliminated or dissipated in models 2 and/or 3, then we will know not only that model 1 was misspecified, but also precisely how the misspecification in model 1 would adversely affect a proper interpretation of the causal nexus of the practice of medicine.

At the most general level, a comparison of the R^2 coefficients for models 1, 2, and 3 (see tables 3.2 and 3.3), yields a considerable amount of support for the general analytic model. Focusing first on modeling the scheduling of routine office visits for new patients (table 3.2), we note that model 1 (the sociodemographic and environmental characteristics) was able to explain 11.7 percent of the variance in the amount of time it takes to schedule a routine office visit for a new patient. When the attitudinal characteristics are added into the equation in model 2, the explained variance increases to 13.8 percent, demonstrating a significant increase in explanatory power, which is consistent with the statistically significant effects of several of the attitudinal measures which we shall discuss shortly. Most important for our theory, however, is the marked increase in explanatory power obtained in model 3, which adds in the practice setting characteristics. The explained variance in model 3 rises to 19.3 percent, which represents an increase in predictive power of approximately 40 percent (as reflected in the statistically significant coefficients for the various practice settings which will be discussed below).

Similarly, when the hierarchical modeling procedure is used to predict the amount of time it takes to schedule routine office visits for an established patient, this pattern is repeated. The R^2 coefficients shown in table 3.3 indicate that when the sociodemographic and environmental characteristics are used to predict scheduling queues for established patients in model 1, 13.0 percent of the variance is explained. When the attitudinal characteristics are included in model 2, the explained variance rises to 14.5 percent. Most importantly, when the practice setting characteristics are added into the equation in model 3, the explained variance rises to 20.7 percent, representing an increase in explanatory power of approximately 43 percent (which is also reflected in the numerous significant coefficients for the practice settings). Overall, then, the comparisons of the R^2 coefficients from models 1, 2, and 3 indicate that (1) the inclusion of the attitudinal characteristics in model 2 does significantly increase the amount of explained variance, although this increase is relatively modest, and (2) the inclusion of the practice setting characteristics in model 3 significantly increases the explanatory power of the general analytic model, on the order of a 40 percent increment in the R^2 levels.

We now focus our attention on the effects of the sociodemographic, environmental, attitudinal, and practice setting characteristics themselves, as reflected in the regression coefficients obtained for them in models 1, 2, and 3. With regard to the effects of these characteristics on the amount of time it takes to schedule routine office visits for new patients, table 3.2 reveals the following. Among the sociodemographic characteristics, sex, AMA membership, board certification, internal medicine, pediatrics, and obstetrics/gynecology all have significant effects, all of which are maintained from model 1 to model 2 to model 3. That is, the introduction of the attitudinal and practice setting characteristics does not annul the effects of the sociodemographic characteristics, although there is some diminution or reduction in the magnitude of the effects of these characteristics. Basically, the effects of the sociodemographic characteristics are as follows. Patients of female physicians have to wait longer to schedule routine office visits than do patients of male physicians. Patients whose physicians are members of the AMA or who are board certified also have to wait longer for an appointment than other patients. The experience of the physician (i.e., the number of years since the M.D. was received), however, was not found to be related to scheduling queues for routine office visits for new patients.

The significance of the specialty dummies (i.e., the effects of internal medicine, pediatrics, and obstetrics/gynecology) shows the importance of controlling for case-mix variation when assessing the amount of time it takes to schedule routine office visits with physicians. These coefficients indicate that it takes the shortest amount of time for a general or family practitioner, and the longest amount of time for an obstetrician/gynecologist, with an internist or a pediatrician falling somewhere in between. (The queues for the internists are slightly longer than those for the pediatricians.) The fact that it is easiest to schedule appointments with general or family practitioners is consistent with Freidson's (1970) theory, which identifies generalists as far more client dependent than specialists; similarly, consistent with Freidson's theory is the fact that it is most difficult to schedule appointments with obstetrician/gynecologists.

Turning to the environmental characteristics, two points are interesting. First, the western United States variable and the physician-to-population ratio never produced a significant effect on scheduling routine office visits for new patients

Table 3.2 Partial regression and R^2 coefficients, T-ratios, and probability levels obtained from the hierarchical modeling of scheduling routine office visits for new patients

	Model 1			Model 2			Model 3		
Variables	b	T-Ratio	Probability Level	b	T-Ratio	Probability Level	b	T-Ratio	Probability Level
Sociodemographic characteristics									
Sex	.217	2.53	.012	.197	2.31	.021	.170	2.06	.039
AMA membership	.096	2.22	.026	.109	2.55	.011	.165	3.93	.000
Board certified	.248	5.58	.000	.216	4.88	.000	.174	4.00	.000
Experience	-.000	-0.18	.854	-.000	-0.07	.944	.003	1.43	.152
Internal medicine	.601	11.94	.000	.606	12.17	.000	.560	11.57	.000
Pediatrics	.491	7.18	.000	.482	7.11	.000	.374	5.65	.000
OB/GYN	.937	15.02	.000	.947	15.30	.000	.899	14.99	.000
Environmental characteristics									
Western U.S.	.084	1.76	.079	.072	1.51	.132	-.071	-1.44	.149
MD/POP ratio	.074	0.58	.559	.052	0.41	.680	-.050	-0.41	.684
Local income	-.092	-3.62	.000	-.090	-3.57	.000	-.108	-4.38	.000
Local education	.107	2.73	.006	.105	2.69	.007	.116	3.07	.002
Attitudinal characteristics									
Business side				-.032	-0.64	.520	-.056	-1.15	.249
Scheduling ease				.172	3.80	.000	.095	2.14	.032
Personal autonomy				-.257	-6.17	.000	-.102	-2.39	.017
Practice location				-.023	0.51	.612	.009	0.20	.844
Earnings potential				-.221	-3.62	.000	-.185	-3.11	.002
Practice setting characteristics									
Kaiser HMO							1.227	10.50	.000
Non-Kaiser group HMO							.534	4.69	.000
Staff HMO							.368	3.12	.002
IPA HMO							.014	0.27	.784
Solo F-F-S							-.291	-6.46	.000
Intercept	.092			.240			.236		
R^2	.117	34.84	.000	.138	28.84	.000	.193	32.86	.000

Table 3.3 Partial regression and R^2 coefficients, *T*-ratios, and probability levels obtained from the hierarchical modeling of scheduling routine office visits for established patients

Variables	Model 1			Model 2			Model 3		
	b	*T- Ratio*	*Probability Level*	b	*T- Ratio*	*Probability Level*	b	*T- Ratio*	*Probability Level*
Sociodemographic characteristics									
Sex	.193	2.24	.025	.174	2.03	.043	.144	1.74	.083
AMA membership	-.027	-0.62	.535	-.014	-0.03	.748	.034	0.80	.424
Board certified	.214	4.75	.000	.190	4.25	.000	.138	3.15	.002
Experience	.001	0.60	.548	.001	0.74	.457	.005	2.47	.014
Internal medicine	.235	4.59	.000	.238	4.69	.000	.185	3.75	.000
Pediatrics	.516	7.22	.000	.504	7.11	.000	.372	5.38	.000
OB/GYN	.987	16.11	.000	.999	16.36	.000	.948	16.08	.000
Environmental characteristics									
Western U.S.	.040	0.83	.405	.030	0.63	.526	-.125	-2.52	.012
MD/POP ratio	.228	1.80	.072	.221	1.76	.079	.130	1.07	.287
Local income	-.059	-2.26	.024	-.058	-2.24	.026	-.077	-3.08	.002
Local education	.076	1.88	.060	.075	1.88	.060	.084	2.19	.028
Attitudinal characteristics									
Business side				-.039	-0.75	.453	-.068	-1.37	.170
Scheduling ease				.138	3.02	.003	.062	1.40	.163
Personal autonomy				-.233	-5.54	.000	-.075	-1.75	.081
Practice location				.008	0.19	.852	-.006	-0.15	.884
Earnings potential				-.103	-1.64	.100	-.006	-1.08	.280
Practice setting characteristics									
Kaiser HMO							1.089	9.74	.000
Non-Kaiser group HMO							.565	5.08	.000
Staff HMO							.348	2.93	.003
IPA HMO							.090	1.70	.090
Solo F-F-S							-.329	-7.24	.000
Intercept	-.001			.103			.135		
R^2	.130	34.45	.000	.145	26.80	.000	.207	31.34	.000

in any of the three models. The western United States variable indicates that pa-tient queues for new patients are no different on the west coast than they are for the rest of the country. Thus, there is no discernible regional variation in pa-tient queues. The absence of an effect of the physician-to-population ratio is somewhat more puzzling. On the one hand, we expected a negative effect such that the greater the supply of physicians (and hence competition among them for patients), the shorter the patient queues. On the other hand, given that the physician-to-population ratios are calculated at the county level, they may well embody sufficient measurement error to prohibit the identification of a statistically significant effect. That is, by using data aggregated across numerous individual physician's areal markets, the relationship between local competition and patient queues may have been obscured (see Mechanic 1979).

The second point among the environmental characteristics that holds across all three models is the significant negative effect of local income and the signifi-cant positive effect of local educational levels on the amount of time it takes to schedule a routine office visit for new patients. The effect of the local income measure is clearly intuitive. That is, the higher the local average income, the lower the patient queue is likely to be. This suggests that physicians are sensitive to the socioeconomic status of their patients, and at least at the aggregate level, they provide shorter patient queues in higher income marketplaces. The positive effect of local median educational level is not so clear. It may indicate that more educated patients have greater scheduling problems of their own which result in longer scheduling queues. It may also indicate that more educated patients, who are more likely to be seeing physicians for routine and preventive services on a regular basis, are better able to accept longer patient queues then less educated patients, who may need more restorative health care (even when scheduling routine office visits).

The effect of the attitudinal characteristics on scheduling queues for new patients focuses on the positive effect of scheduling ease and the negative effects of personal autonomy and earnings potential. The scheduling ease and earnings potential effects are basically the same in model 2 and model 3, although the effect of personal autonomy is significantly diminished in model 3 by the introduction of the practice setting characteristics. Patients of physicians who indicated that scheduling ease was very important in their selection of a practice setting have to wait longer to schedule an appointment than do their counterparts who see physicians who do not feel that scheduling ease is as important. This is as expected and simply indicates that for physicians for whom scheduling ease is an important issue, scheduling queues are longer. Similarly, the negative effect of earnings poten-tial on patient queues is also as anticipated. That is, for physicians who find earn-ings potential important in selecting a practice setting, patient queues are signif-icantly shorter, reflecting their attention to patient dependency as a means of ensuring the earnings potential of their practice. Finally, the negative effect of personal autonomy is also as expected. Physicians for whom the personal autonomy issue was very important in selecting a practice setting have significantly shorter patient queues. This reflects their greater patient dependency and, perhaps, their closer relationships with their patients. As indicated earlier, however, the overall effect of the attitudinal characteristics on new patient scheduling queues is not great.

Turning to the effects of the practice setting characteristics, we find that the results are perfectly consistent with our theory. That is, our theory suggests that patient queues should be arrayed from the longest to the shortest in the following order: Kaiser model HMOs, non-Kaiser group model HMOs, staff model HMOs, IPA model HMOs, group fee-for-service practices, and solo fee-for-service practices. The regression coefficients obtained from model 3 fit this hierarchical sequence precisely. The IPA model physicians impose patient queues not significantly different from their group fee-for-service counterparts, as we expected. Moreover, as indicated earlier, the addition of the practice setting characteristics to model 3 increases the explanatory power of the general analytic model by about 40 percent. Thus, the data in table 3.2 provide considerable support for the general analytic model, as well as for the particular predictions of our theory in terms of the patient queues associated with the various practice settings.

The results obtained from models 1, 2, and 3 in predicting the scheduling of office visits for established patients are very similar to those for new patients. At the general level, the R^2 coefficients obtained for established patients are very similar for all three models to those obtained for new patients. The effects for the four sets of characteristics (the sociodemographic, environmental, attitudinal, and practice setting characteristics) obtained when modeling the scheduling of routine visits for established patients are also similar to those obtained from modeling the scheduling of routine office visits for new patients, although there are some differences. We shall focus here on the differences.

Among the sociodemographic characteristics, only AMA membership fails to produce statistically significant results with respect to established patient queues. Established patients of female physicians and board certified physicians again have longer patient queues. For established patients, the experience of the physician produces a significant positive effect, but only in model 3. This indicates that when practice settings are taken into consideration, patients who see older (i.e., more experienced) physicians have to wait longer than patients who see younger physicians.

The effects of the set of dummy variables for medical specialty are quite similar for established patients and new patients, with one exception. For established patients, the queue is shorter for internists than for pediatricians, the reverse of what we found for new patients. Thus, for established patients the shortest queue is for those seeing general or family practitioners, followed by a slightly longer queue for those seeing internists, followed by an even longer queue for those seeing pediatricians, with the longest queue for those who are seeing obstetrician/gynecologists.

Two points warrant further discussion. The significantly longer time period necessary for a new as opposed to an established patient to schedule an appointment with an internist may indicate that internists provide more extensive diagnostic services in their offices on a consulting or referral basis. Thus, they may be more willing to satisfy their established patients by minimizing their appointment scheduling time, as opposed to the considerably longer queues that they impose upon new patients, who are primarily referrals and who are not likely to return. Quite to the contrary, the relative consistency between the patient queues imposed upon new and established patients by pediatricians and obstetrician/gynecologists indicates that they provide relatively few consultative services, with most of their new patients becoming ongoing patients.

As indicated in table 3.3, the effect of the environmental characteristics on patient queues for established patients is virtually the same as for new patients. The one exception involves the effect of the western United States variable. When the practice setting characteristics are introduced in model 3, the negative effect of the western United States variable becomes significant. While this is not necessarily straightforward, it may indicate that in the western United States, where competition among physicians is generally greater and where innovations in medical practice typically occur first, physicians may be somewhat more patient dependent. This interpretation, however, is at best speculative, because the negative effect of the western United States variable occurs only in model 3, and because the physician-to-population ratio fails to indicate any significant effect of competition. The significant negative effect of income and the significant positive effect of local education on established patient scheduling queues are very similar to those found in table 3.2. Again, where income is higher, patient queues are shorter; where education is higher, patient queues are longer.

When the attitudinal characteristics are first introduced in model 2, their effects for established patients are nearly identical to those for new patients. That is, in model 2 a statistically significant positive effect is found for scheduling ease, while statistically significant negative effects are found for personal autonomy and earnings potential. Our interpretation of these effects on established patients is the same as it was for new patients. Physicians for whom scheduling ease is a very important issue in selecting a practice setting impose longer patient queues on their established patients than do their counterparts. Similarly, physicians whose attitudes reflect greater client dependency (i.e., who view personal autonomy and earnings potential as very important) impose shorter queues on their established patients. However, when the practice setting characteristics are introduced in model 3, the effects of the attitudinal characteristics are reduced to the point of spuriousness. That is, none of the attitudinal characteristics produces a statistically significant effect in model 3. Thus, what was recognized in model 2 as a nature effect is recognized as a nurture effect in model 3.

Turning to the practice setting characteristics that are introduced in model 3, we see the same pattern for established patients as for new patients. Once again, all of the coefficients for the set of dummy variables measuring the practice settings (except IPA model HMOs) are statistically significant. Moreover, the ordering of the practice settings in terms of the patient queues imposed on established patients is, from the longest queue to the shortest queue, as follows: Kaiser model HMOs, non-Kaiser group model HMOs, staff model HMOs, IPA model HMOs, group fee-for-service practices, and solo fee-for-service practices. Moreover, the effect of the IPA model HMO practice setting variable again is not significant, just as our theory predicted. That is, scheduling queues for established patients in IPA model HMOs are not statistically different from those in group fee-for-service practices. Thus, the data in table 3.3 provide considerable further support for our theory.

Table 3.4 contains the results of the hierarchical application of the general analytic model to waiting time on arrival for a scheduled appointment. An initial comparison of the partial regression and R^2 coefficients shown in table 3.4 with those shown in tables 3.2 and 3.3 suggests that patient scheduling queues and waiting times are, indeed, distinct phenomena having distinct determinant structures. For example, while the general analytic model works rather well in predicting the amount of time necessary for both new and established patients to schedule a routine office visit ($R^2 = .193$ and $.207$, respectively), the model does not work well in explaining the amount of time that patients must subsequently wait in the physician's office ($R^2 = .061$). Moreover, while the signs and magnitudes of the regression coefficients for the four sets of characteristics are consistent for the new and established patient scheduling queues, the signs of these coefficients are often reversed when predicting waiting time upon arrival for the scheduled appointment. Thus, we conclude that the determinants of office waiting time are, in fact, different from the determinants of scheduling queues.

Among the sociodemographic characteristics, only the set of specialty dummies and the experience variable produced statistically significant effects on office waiting times across all three models. Patients who have female physicians face the same office waiting times as patients of male physicians. Patients whose physicians are members of the AMA have slightly longer office waits, although this significant difference almost disappears when the practice setting characteristics are introduced in model 3. Patients who see board certified physicians have waiting room queues similar to patients who see non-board certified physicians. Patients who see more experienced (i.e., older) physicians generally have shorter waiting room queues. This probably reflects the phenomenon that younger physicians are more likely to see walk-in and emergency patients than are their seniors, who are more likely to have established ongoing relationships with their patients, and who see them more frequently for routine visits. Therefore younger physicians

Table 3.4 Partial regression and R^2 coefficients, T-ratios, and probability levels obtained from the hierarchical modeling of waiting time on arrival for scheduled appointments

Variables	Model 1			Model 2			Model 3		
	b	T-Ratio	Probability Level	b	T-Ratio	Probability Level	b	T-Ratio	Probability Level
Sociodemographic characteristics									
Sex	-.042	-0.84	.402	-.034	-0.68	.498	-.033	-0.67	.501
AMA membership	.062	2.57	.010	.058	2.40	.017	.048	1.94	.052
Board certified	.014	0.58	.563	.017	0.70	.486	-.003	-0.13	.894
Experience	-.004	-3.74	.000	-.004	-4.02	.000	-.003	-3.07	.002
Internal medicine	-.204	-7.27	.000	-.204	-7.28	.000	-.208	-7.43	.000
Pediatrics	-.125	-3.41	.001	-.126	-3.46	.001	-.137	-3.74	.000
OB/GYN	-.013	-0.37	.709	-.008	-0.21	.831	-.011	-0.32	.749
Environmental characteristics									
Western U.S.	-.075	-2.78	.006	-.070	-2.59	.010	-.060	-2.11	.035
MD/POP ratio	-.000	-0.00	.998	.007	0.10	.920	.013	0.18	.857
Local income	-.022	-1.54	.123	-.022	-1.52	.129	-.017	-1.21	.227
Local education	-.072	-3.35	.001	-.073	-3.39	.001	-.076	-3.56	.000
Attitudinal characteristics									
Business side				-.005	-0.16	.874	-.007	-0.25	.804
Scheduling ease				-.085	-3.31	.001	-.096	-3.72	.000
Personal autonomy				-.029	-1.24	.214	.002	0.08	.940
Practice location				-.048	-1.90	.057	-.047	-1.87	.062
Earnings potential				.059	1.72	.086	.056	1.62	.106
Practice setting characteristics									
Kaiser HMO							-.154	-2.15	.031
Non-Kaiser group HMO							-.162	-2.39	.017
Staff HMO							-.076	-1.06	.291
IPA HMO							-.024	-0.79	.431
Solo F-F-S							-.132	-5.08	.000
Intercept	4.002			4.067			4.147		
R^2	.046	14.51	.000	.052	11.32	.000	.061	10.20	.000

devote a larger proportion of their practice to emergency situations or nonroutine visits and should thus experience more stochastic scheduling shocks, resulting in longer waiting room queues.

The effects of the medical specialty characteristics on the amount of time patients spend in the office upon arriving for the scheduled appointment illustrates the difference between this type of patient queue and that involved in scheduling. While all three medical specialty dummies produced significant positive effects on the scheduling of appointments, they produced significant (except for obstetrics/gynecology) negative effects on patient queues in the office. This means that after arriving for scheduled routine visits, patients must wait longer to see general or family practitioners than to see internists, pediatricians, or obstetrician/gynecologists. Nonetheless, these data are generally consistent with the previous findings concerning appointment scheduling. Most primary care specialists' patients are likely to be either scheduled referrals or scheduled ongoing patients. The client-dependent practice of the general or family practitioner, however, is more subject to the stochastic shock of unscheduled and emergency cases. Thus, waiting times for the patients of general or family practitioners are likely to be longer, regardless of their appointment status.

Among the environmental characteristics, only the western United States and local educational level variables produced significant effects. Patients of physicians practicing in the western United States generally have shorter waiting room queues than in the rest of the country. As indicated earlier, this may reflect the trend-setting role of the west coast in medical practice. That is, innovations in medical practice generally originate on the west coast and are subsequently diffused eastward. In this period of increasing physician competition and consumer awareness, west coast physicians may simply be responding more rapidly to the new situation in health care delivery than their counterparts.

With regard to local median educational levels, the data in table 3.4 indicate that the higher the educational level, the shorter the waiting room queue. Although this effect is the reverse of that which we found for scheduling routine office visits, it is not necessarily inconsistent. As we suggested earlier, it is reasonable to assume that the positive effect of local educational levels on scheduling queues reflects the increased difficulties of more educated patients to fit routine office visits into their own schedule. Once those visits are scheduled, however, more educated patients may be more likely to keep those appointments and arrive on time, thus serving to minimize office waiting room queues.

Among the attitudinal characteristics introduced in model 2, only scheduling ease had a statistically significant effect on waiting room queues. Among physicians who indicate that scheduling ease is a very important issue in selecting a practice setting, waiting room queues are significantly shorter. This probably indicates that those physicians want to minimize waiting room queues in order to improve both their patients' and their own satisfaction. The patient's satisfaction is improved by reducing waiting time; the physician's satisfaction is improved by avoiding crowded waiting rooms and agitated patients who have to wait too long. The effect of scheduling ease on waiting room queues remains even after the practice setting characteristics are introduced in model 3.

Among the practice setting characteristics introduced in model 3, statistically significant negative effects were obtained for Kaiser model HMOs, non-Kaiser model group HMOs, and solo fee-for-service practice settings. The dummy variables for staff model and IPA model HMOs did not yield statistically significant results. Unlike their effects on scheduling queues, which uniformly conformed to our theoretical expectations, the effects of the practice setting characteristics on waiting room queues do not provide as much support for our theory. We did not expect IPA model HMOs to be significantly different from group fee-for-service practice settings, and they are not. We did, however, expect physicians in staff model HMOs to have waiting room queues significantly different from physicians in group fee-for-service settings, but they do not. Finally, we did expect physicians in Kaiser model HMOs, non-Kaiser group model HMOs, and solo fee-for-service practice settings to have waiting room queues significantly different from their group fee-for-service counterparts, and they do. However, the direction of those significant differences are not all as we expected. Solo fee-for-service physicians do have significantly shorter waiting room queues than those in group fee-for-service, just as we expected. Kaiser model HMO and non-Kaiser group model HMO physicians, however, also have significantly shorter waiting room queues than fee-for-service group practice physicians. This is not consistent with our theory.

Moreover, the magnitude of the coefficients for the solo fee-for-service, Kaiser model HMO, and non-Kaiser group model HMO variables suggests that in these three practice settings patients wait about the same amount of time in the office. This, of course, appears anomalous given extant presuppositions (see Held and Reinhardt 1979). What these data may actually indicate is an explicit attempt by physicians in Kaiser and non-Kaiser group model HMOs to offset the "clinic" atmosphere generally attributed to their medical practice form (see Berki and Ashcraft 1980). To do this, these physicians may concentrate on reducing waiting room queues in order to improve their public image and create the impression of providing medical care (in terms of waiting room times) that is indistinguishable from that found in solo fee-for-service practices. Thus, although the effects of the practice setting characteristics on waiting room queues are not exactly as we had expected, the pattern of effects is both plausible and understandable.

At this point the reader might ask whether or not waiting room queues depend in part on the volume of patients seen, such that patients of busier physicians have to wait longer than patients of less busy physicians. We have chosen not to include the volume of patients in the general analytic model for three reasons. First, it has not been included in previous studies, although its inclusion would seem straightforward. Second, it is directly applicable only to modeling waiting room queues, and including it would detract from the flow of applying the same general analytic model to all of the measures of how medicine is practiced. Third, including the volume of patients does not alter our results. Although the volume of patients has a significant positive effect on waiting room queues and increases the explained variance, the effects of the practice setting and other characteristics remain the same. Therefore, we report only on the results of the general analytic model.

Although tables 3.2, 3.3, and 3.4 present the precise effects on patient queues for each of the variables in our general analytic model, they do not intuitively portray the magnitude of the differences in patient queues across the various organizational forms of medical practice. To compensate for these shortcomings, we used the precise effects of the general analytic model to adjust new and established patient scheduling and waiting room queues within each of the six practice settings for differences in the sociodemographic, environmental, and attitudinal characteristics. Our adjustment procedure statistically removes these differences. Table 3.5 shows the results of these calculations. As the numbers in table 3.5 indicate, the differences in the average adjusted patient queues for physicians in the various practice settings are quite consistent (except for waiting room queues) with our original theoretical expectations, which were graphically displayed in figure 1.5. Thus the data in table 3.5 flesh out a more intuitively pleasing demonstration of the support for our theory than can be obtained solely from the hierarchical regression results presented in tables 3.2, 3.3 and 3.4.

The Organization of Medical Practice and Time Spent with Patients

The amount of time spent per patient in the office (and in the hospital) was calculated by dividing the number of hours practiced in the office (hospital) by the number of patients seen in the office (hospital). Although the actual numbers of minutes are reported in table 3.1, the natural logarithms of the average numbers of minutes are used in the hierarchical modeling (see tables 3.6 and 3.7).

These data indicate that the general analytic model is not as robust in predicting the amount of time spent with patients as it is in predicting patient queues. For example, although the general analytic model is able to explain about 20 percent of the variance in scheduling queues, the explained variance for the time spent with patients in the office is only 15.3 percent, and for the amount of time spent with patients in the hospital it is only 7.5 percent. It would appear that the amount of time spent with patients is not as much a function of the sociodemographic, environmental, attitudinal, and practice setting characteristics as are patient queues.

Table 3.5   Average adjusted means for the patient queues by practice
             setting

		Scheduling Queues	
Practice Setting	*New Patients*	*Established Patients*	*Waiting Room Queues*
Kaiser model HMO	17.9	9.6	16.5
Non-Kaiser group model HMO	8.9	5.7	16.3
Staff model HMO	7.6	4.6	17.8
IPA model HMO	5.3	3.5	18.7
Group fee-for-service	5.2	3.2	19.2
Solo fee-for-service	3.9	2.3	16.8

Note: Means are adjusted for the effects of the sociodemographic, environmental, and attitudinal characteristics. Scheduling queues are shown in actual number of days, and waiting room queues in actual number of minutes.

Moreover, in the analysis of the patient queues data there were considerable increments in the level of explained variance between models 1 and 2 and between models 2 and 3. This is not the case with time spent with patients. Indeed, the difference in explained variance between model 1 and model 3 for the amount of time spent per patient in the office is but 0.8 percent; the difference is only 2.0 percent for the amount of time spent per patient in the hospital. Thus, the attitudinal and practice setting characteristics introduced in models 2 and 3 contribute little new information to explain the variance in the amount of time spent with patients. Finally, the difference between the explained variance levels obtained for the amount of time spent with patients in the office versus the hospital (i.e., 15.3 percent versus 7.5 percent) indicates that average office visit lengths are more a function of the sociodemographic, environmental, attitudinal, and practice setting characteristics than are average hospital visit lengths. Accordingly, we shall discuss the individual regression coefficients separately for time spent per patient in the office and in the hospital.

For time spent per patient in the office (table 3.6), all of the sociodemographic characteristics (except the dummy variables for pediatricians and obstetrician/gynecologists) produce statistically significant effects. The average length of an office visit for patients who see female physicians is longer than for patients who see male physicians. This may help to explain why female physician incomes are generally lower than male physician incomes; if female physicians are spending more time per patient in the office, then they can see fewer patients per hour, and they generate lower revenues than their male counterparts. Physicians who are members of the AMA or who are board certified spend less time per patient in the office than those who are not AMA members and not board certified. This

Table 3.6 Partial regression and R^2 coefficients, T-ratios, and probability levels obtained from the hierarchical modeling of the amount of time spent per patient in the office

Variables	Model 1			Model 2			Model 3		
	b	T-Ratio	Probability Level	b	T-Ratio	Probability Level	b	T-Ratio	Probability Level
Sociodemographic characteristics									
Sex	.175	4.52	.000	.174	4.49	.000	.180	4.67	.000
AMA membership	-.076	-4.02	.000	-.074	-3.94	.000	-.080	-4.22	.000
Board certified	-.047	-2.45	.015	-.045	-2.34	.020	-.038	-1.94	.053
Experience	.002	2.97	.003	.002	2.68	.007	.002	2.15	.032
Internal medicine	.317	14.62	.000	.314	14.52	.000	.323	14.91	.000
Pediatrics	-.053	-1.86	.064	-.051	-1.78	.075	-.033	-1.16	.248
OB/GYN	-.029	-1.05	.292	-.029	-1.03	.302	-.021	-0.75	.455
Environmental characteristics									
Western U.S.	.044	2.08	.037	.044	2.11	.035	.072	3.23	.001
MD/POP ratio	.366	6.64	.000	.365	6.62	.000	.378	6.82	.000
Local income	.022	2.01	.045	.022	2.02	.044	.024	2.17	.030
Local education	.047	2.88	.004	.047	2.85	.004	.046	2.85	.005
Attitudinal characteristics									
Business side				-.021	-0.96	.337	-.017	-0.77	.442
Scheduling ease				.003	0.14	.886	.013	0.67	.503
Personal autonomy				.039	2.11	.035	.015	0.79	.431
Practice location				-.003	-0.17	.862	-.001	-0.09	.928
Earnings potential				-.038	-1.43	.153	-.041	-1.55	.121
Practice setting characteristics									
Kaiser HMO							-.209	-3.79	.000
Non-Kaiser group HMO							-.120	-2.30	.022
Staff HMO							.005	0.09	.926
IPA HMO							-.031	-1.30	.195
Solo F-F-S							.041	2.02	.044
Intercept	2.220			2.218			2.207		
R^2	.145	51.54	.000	.147	35.96	.000	.153	28.81	.000

Table 3.7 Partial regression and R^2 coefficients, T-ratios, and probability levels obtained from the hierarchical modeling of the amount of time spent per patient in the hospital

Variables	Model 1			Model 2			Model 3		
	b	T-Ratio	Probability Level	b	T-Ratio	Probability Level	b	T-Ratio	Probability Level
Sociodemographic characteristics									
Sex	.149	2.18	.029	.147	2.15	.032	.146	2.16	.031
AMA membership	-.105	-3.42	.001	-.106	-3.47	.001	-.102	-3.31	.001
Board certified	-.125	-4.01	.000	-.126	-4.01	.000	-.097	-3.07	.002
Experience	-.002	-1.30	.195	-.002	-1.45	.149	-.003	-2.31	.021
Internal medicine	-.009	-0.26	.791	-.011	-0.31	.756	.002	0.05	.959
Pediatrics	.127	2.74	.006	.131	2.84	.005	.162	3.49	.001
OB/GYN	.365	8.13	.000	.371	8.26	.000	.382	8.53	.000
Environmental characteristics									
Western U.S.	.058	1.70	.089	.052	1.50	.133	.064	1.78	.075
MD/POP ratio	.291	3.19	.001	.291	3.19	.001	.277	3.03	.003
Local income	-.029	-1.65	.099	-.027	-1.50	.135	-.030	-1.67	.094
Local education	.113	4.25	.000	.109	4.12	.000	.113	4.28	.000
Attitudinal characteristics									
Business side				-.013	-0.37	.714	-.004	-0.11	.916
Scheduling ease				-.057	-1.78	.075	-.034	-1.05	.292
Personal autonomy				.041	1.40	.162	-.012	-0.39	.696
Practice location				.070	2.19	.028	.070	2.23	.026
Earnings potential				-.079	-1.82	.069	-.078	-1.81	.071
Practice setting characteristics									
Kaiser HMO							-.149	-1.59	.113
Non-Kaiser group HMO							.141	1.54	.125
Staff HMO							.307	3.34	.001
IPA HMO							.012	0.33	.745
Solo F-F-S							.187	5.76	.000
Intercept	2.330			2.350			2.241		
R^2	.055	15.99	.000	.060	11.86	.000	.075	11.52	.000

may indicate that these physicians do more consultative work, which may require shorter visits, given that the preliminary workup for the patient has already been done by the referring physician. Those with more experience spend slightly more time with their patients in the office than their less experienced colleagues, although this difference is not great. The largest effect of the sociodemographic characteristics on the amount of time spent per patient in the office is that of the dummy variable for internal medicine. Internists spend considerably more time (approximately ten minutes more) with each of their patients than general or family practitioners. This probably reflects the fact that internists provide more extensive diagnostic services in their offices, compared with the briefer services of their general or family practice, pediatrician, or obstetrician/gynecologist counterparts.

At this point, it is important to note that the effects of the sociodemographic characteristics on the amount of time spent per patient in the office are relatively constant across all three models. That is, these effects are neither made spurious nor are they significantly diminished by the introduction of either the attitudinal or practice setting characteristics. This indicates that the sociodemographic characteristics of physicians are quite important in determining the amount of time they will spend per patient in the office setting.

Similarly, the data in table 3.6 indicate that all four of the environmental characteristics have statistically significant effects on the amount of time spent per patient in the office and that the magnitude of these effects remains virtually the same across all three regression models. Physicians who practice in the western United States spend more time with their patients in the office than their counterparts in other areas of the country. This again may reflect the innovative characteristics of west coast physicians as part of their response to changes in the health care delivery system; that is, west coast physicians may be spending more time per patient in order to maintain their patient loads in the face of the changing health care delivery system. Similarly, physicians who are practicing in areas with higher physician-to-population ratios also spend more time in the office with their patients. This may be interpreted as a direct indication of physicians' responses to increasing competition. As competition for patients increases, more time will be spent with each patient in order to maintain that patient within the practice.

Both measures of the local patient pool (i.e., local income and educational levels) also produced positive effects on the amount of time spent with patients in the office. The higher the local income and educational levels, the longer the office visit. This may indicate that physicians and other health care providers are now paying special attention to patients who have sufficient financial resources (whether in terms of third-party insurance or personal assets) to pay for the services that they consume. In these changing reimbursement times, physicians and other providers may be giving special attention (i.e., spending more time) to patients for whom reimbursement is not viewed as problematic. When taken together, the environmental characteristics clearly indicate that the practice of medicine is quite sensitive to the environment of the areal marketplace.

When the attitudinal characteristics are introduced in model 2, only personal autonomy produces a significant effect on the amount of time spent per patient in the office. As expected, this effect is positive and indicates that physicians for whom personal autonomy is very important in selecting a practice setting spend more time with their patients. Because a desire for personal autonomy in a practice setting reflects a willingness to accept client dependency rather than colleague dependency, longer office visits among physicians who prefer to be client-dependent are not surprising. When the practice setting characteristics are introduced in model 3, however, the positive effect of personal autonomy is reduced to insignificance, indicating that the effect demonstrated in model 2 was spurious.

The effect of the practice setting characteristics introduced in model 3 on the amount of time spent per patient in the office is almost exactly what our theory had suggested. Physicians in solo fee-for-service practice have the longest patient visits, followed in order by physicians in group fee-for-service practice, IPA model HMOs, staff model HMOs, and non-Kaiser group model HMOs, with Kaiser model HMO physicians having the shortest office visit lengths of all. Moreover, as our theory states, office visit lengths among IPA model HMO physicians are not significantly different from those among group fee-for-service physicians. The only divergent finding here is the effect of staff model HMO physicians. Our theory suggests that staff model HMO physicians will have significantly shorter average office visit lengths than group fee-for-service physicians. However, the regression coefficient obtained from model 3 indicates that the average office visit length of staff model HMO physicians is not statistically significantly different from that of group fee-for-service physicians.

In spite of these variations from expectations, the results reported in table 3.5 provide considerable support for our theory, as well as for the previous work of Mechanic (1975) and Freidson (1970). The consistently greater amounts of time spent by physicians at the solo end of the autonomous versus bureaucratic dimension of medical practice reflects a greater sense of client dependency, in contrast with the greater colleague dependency felt by physicians at the other end of the continuum. In the more autonomous practice settings physicians depend more directly on patients for patient flow (especially in general or family practice) than their counterparts who have joined together in some form of collaborative practice arrangement. The latter may receive patients through the secondary benefit of the brand name effect of the group, or on direct referral from their partners; physicians in solo practice do not enjoy such advantages. Moreover, the "real" source of patients in the HMO settings is not the patients themselves, but the employer groups who provide the HMO option to their employees.

The effects of the general analytic model on the amount of time spent per patient in the hospital show somewhat different patterns (see table 3.7). Among the sociodemographic characteristics, only internal medicine fails to produce a significant effect on the amount of time spent in the hospital. (It had been the most significant predictor of the amount of time spent in the office.) Again, female physicians spend more time per patient in the hospital than do males, and physicians who are members of the AMA or who are board certified spend less than their counterparts. The effect of experience on the amount of time spent per patient in the hospital is negative, the reverse of what it was in the office setting. On the one hand, this negative effect may indicate that more experienced physicians simply need to spend less time with their hospitalized patients than less experienced physicians. On the other hand, the positive effect of experience on the amount of time spent per patient in the office may indicate that more experienced physicians spend more time with their patients in the office in order to arrive at the most appropriate diagnosis. Further study, however, is necessary before these interpretations can be considered more than speculative. Perhaps the ambiguity of a "hospital visit" introduces significant measurement error into the results.

Of the sociodemographic characteristics, internal medicine has the most interesting effect (actually, noneffect) on the amount of time spent per patient in the hospital. That the coefficient for internal medicine on the length of hospital visits measure is not significant suggests that internists provide more extensive diagnostic services in their offices compared with more brief consultative services in the hospital. Pediatricians and obstetrician/gynecologists, in contrast, spend significantly more time than general or family practitioners with their hospitalized patients, although they spend about the same amount of time as general or family practitioners with their office patients. This probably reflects the greater hospital or surgical orientation of pediatricians and obstetrician/gynecologists when compared with general or family practitioners.

Among the environmental characteristics, the western United States variable and the local income measure failed to produce statistically significant effects on the amount of time spent per patient in the hospital. The effects of the physician-to-population ratio and the local median educational level are both positive and statistically significant. The positive effect of the physician-to-population ratio once again suggests that in the face of increasing competition (i.e., higher ratios), physicians will spend more time with their patients in an attempt to maintain those patients within their practices. Similarly, the positive effect of the local median educational level is also consistent with that found for the amount of time spent per patient in the office. It probably reflects special considerations given to patients who are better reimbursement candidates than less educated patients.

When the attitudinal characteristics are introduced in model 2, only the practice location measure produces a statistically significant effect. Physicians for whom location is very important in selecting a practice setting spend more time with their patients in the hospital. This practice location effect is not diminished when the practice setting characteristics are introduced in model 3. The effect of practice location may be a proxy for the convenience of a practice setting in terms of minimizing travel time to hospitals. As a result of minimized travel time, these physicians may be able to spend more time with their patients in the hospital.

Turning to the effects of the practice setting characteristics, the results indicate that our theory is not as well supported for hospital visit lengths as it was for office visit lengths. Indeed, only the staff model HMO and the solo fee-for-service variables produced statistically significant effects. The regression coefficients indicate that solo fee-for-service physicians spend more time per patient in the hospital than do group fee-for-service physicians. However, the regression coefficients also indicate that staff model HMO physicians spend even more time than do solo fee-for-service physicians. The rather anomalous effect of the staff model HMO physicians may reflect the fact that they are generally salaried employees and have less of a proprietary interest in generating practice incomes than either their solo or group fee-for-service counterparts.

As expected, the hospital visit lengths of IPA model HMO physicians are no different from those of their group fee-for-service practice counterparts. Also as expected, although not statistically significant, is the fact that Kaiser model HMO physicians spend the smallest amount of time with their patients in the hospital. This is consistent with our general theory, and supports Mechanic's (1975) argument that group model HMO physicians will respond to increasing patient demands by spending less time per patient.

Although neither the Kaiser model HMO nor the non-Kaiser group model HMO coefficients are statistically significant, they are of different signs. The effect of the Kaiser model HMO is negative, while the effect of the non-Kaiser group model HMO is positive, both approaching statistical significance. This underscores the importance of distinguishing between the traditional Kaiser model HMOs and the new hybrid FFS/PPD groups identified by Krill and Gaynor (1982). Indeed, the magnitude of the difference between these regression coefficients (when compared with the group fee-for-service category) indicates that these two HMO types are significantly different from each other, although not significantly different from group fee-for-service practice settings.

Although the results shown for the practice setting characteristics in table 3.7 do not support our theory as uniformly as the results contained in table 3.6, they do provide some evidence. The difference between the support demonstrated for our theory in tables 3.6 and 3.7 suggests that practice settings are more important for office visits than for hospital visits. Perhaps hospital visits are more standardized or uniform than office visits. It is also obvious that office practice settings are more important to office visit lengths than to hospital visit lengths, because for the latter, the particular configuration of the office practice may not be terribly relevant.

Although tables 3.6 and 3.7 present the precise effects on the amount of time spent with patients for each of the variables in our general analytic model, they do not intuitively portray the magnitude of the differences in the amount of time spent with patients across the various practice settings. To compensate for these shortcomings, we again used the precise effects of the general analytic model to adjust the average amount of time that physicians spend with their patients in the office and in the hospital within each of the six practice settings for differences in the sociodemographic, environmental, and attitudinal characteristics. The results of these calculations are shown in table 3.8. The adjusted average amounts of time spent with patients in the office are quite consistent with our theoretical expectations, which were graphically portrayed in figure 1.5. The adjusted average amounts of time spent with patients in the hospital, however, are not as consistent with our theoretical expectations. Again, this indicates that the effect of the practice setting on how much time is spent with patients in the hospital is not as straightforward as it is in the office. This is understandable and probably means that constraints on office behavior introduced by the office practice setting simply do not carry over into the hospital practice setting.

Summary and Discussion

A considerable amount of information has been presented from the complex statistical analyses that were reported in this chapter. The best way to summarize and discuss these results is to focus on the six most important points that have emerged about how the organization of medical practice affects the practice of medicine. The first concerns the effect on patient scheduling queues. Our theory had suggested that patient scheduling queues should be arrayed from the longest to the shortest in the following order: Kaiser model HMOs, non-Kaiser group model HMOs, staff model HMOs, IPA model HMOs, group fee-for-service practices, and solo fee-for-service practices. The regression coefficients obtained from model 3 for both of the patient scheduling queues (tables 3.2 and 3.3) fit this ordered sequence precisely. Moreover, the addition of the practice setting characteristics to model 3 increased the explanatory power of the general analytic model by about 40 percent. Thus, the analysis of the patient scheduling queue data provides considerable support for the general analytic model, as well as for the particular predictions of our theory in terms of the patient scheduling queues associated with the various practice settings.

The second point is that the effects of the practice setting characteristics when used to predict waiting room queues were statistically significant but not entirely as we had expected. In particular, statistically significant negative effects were obtained for Kaiser model HMOs, non-Kaiser model group HMOs, and solo

Table 3.8   Average adjusted means of the amount of
time spent with patients by practice setting

Practice Settings	Office Visits	Hospital Visits
Kaiser model HMO	17.6	26.3
Non-Kaiser group model HMO	19.3	35.1
Staff model HMO	21.8	41.5
IPA model HMO	21.1	30.9
Group fee-for-service	21.7	30.5
Solo fee-for-service	22.6	36.8

Note: Means are adjusted for the effects of the sociodemographic, environmental, and attitudinal characteristics. Time spent with patients is shown in the actual number of minutes.

fee-for-service practice settings. Moreover, the magnitude of the coefficients for these three practice settings suggests that patients must wait about the same amount of time on arrival at the office. At first glance, this seems anomalous. Existing theories suggest that in both Kaiser and non-Kaiser group model HMOs, waiting room queues are used as nonprice rationing devices to counter increased patient demand spurred by moral hazard factors. We believe, however, that these data probably reflect the fact that explicit attempts are being made by physicians in Kaiser and non-Kaiser group model HMOs to offset the "clinic" atmosphere generally associated with their medical practice settings. To do this, physicians in these HMO settings may be concentrating on reducing their waiting room queues in order to improve their public image and create the impression of having waiting room queues that are indistinguishable from those found in solo fee-for-service practices. Thus, although the effects of practice settings on waiting room queues are not exactly as our theory would predict, these results can be explained in a reasonable, albeit ad hoc fashion.

The third important point to be noted from these analyses is the fact that patient scheduling and waiting room queues are distinct phenomena having distinct determinant structures. In particular, our general analytic model worked rather well in predicting patient scheduling queues, but not well at all in explaining waiting room queues. Moreover, while the signs and magnitudes of the regression coefficients for the four sets of characteristics (sociodemographic, environmental, attitudinal, and practice setting) were generally consistent for new and established patient scheduling queues, this was not the case for waiting room queues. Indeed, these results suggest that the amount of time patients spend in the waiting room appears to be a more random phenomenon, at least as far as organizational structure and the other characteristics examined herein are concerned. Thus, future structural alterations of the health care delivery system are not likely to affect waiting room queues, although they may have some impact on patient satisfaction with those queues.

Fourth, the effect of the practice setting characteristics on the amount of time spent per patient in the office is almost exactly as our theory had suggested. Indeed, the six practice settings are arrayed as follows, from longest to shortest patient visits: solo fee-for-service practice, group fee-for-service practice, IPA model HMOs, staff model HMOs, non-Kaiser group model HMOs, and Kaiser model HMOs. Indeed, the only result that does not fit perfectly with our theoretical expectations is the fact that while staff model HMO physicians spend less time per patient in the office than do group fee-for-service physicians, this one difference was not statistically significant. These results clearly support our theory, as well as the pioneering work of Freidson (1970), Mechanic (1975), and Held and Reinhardt (1979).

Fifth, unlike the analysis of the office visit lengths (which provided considerable support for our theory), only the staff model HMO and the solo fee-for-service practice settings produced statistically significant effects on hospital visit lengths. As expected, solo fee-for-service physicians spend more time per patient in the hospital than their group fee-for-service counterparts. However, the results indicate that staff model HMO physicians spend even more time per patient in the hospital than either of the other types. Although somewhat anomalous, these results may be explained in an ad hoc fashion. That staff model HMO physicians spend the most time per patient in the hospital may reflect the fact that they are generally salaried employees; thus, they have the least proprietary interest in generating practice incomes. Accordingly, they can afford to spend more time per patient in the hospital. To some extent, additional support for this interpretation is provided by the fact that although the effect of the Kaiser model HMO practice setting was not statistically significant, the results do indicate that Kaiser model HMO physicians spend the smallest amount of time with their patients in the hospital. This is consistent with our theory, as well as Mechanic's (1975), suggesting that group model HMO physicians may respond to increasing patient demands by spending less time per patient.

Sixth, different results were obtained by applying the general analytic model to the amounts of time spent per patient in the office and in the hospital. These differences probably reflect the fact that the office practice setting has a greater effect on the practice of medicine in the office than in the hospital. This is intuitively pleasing, because the office practice setting effect may not "spill over" into the hospital setting, especially if the hospital is neither owned nor controlled by the office medical practice. Further, the difference in the effects of the practice setting characteristics on these amounts of time may also mean that hospital visits are more standardized or uniform. That is, it may be that there is significantly less latitude with which physicians may operate in the hospital than in the office practice setting. Office visit lengths may be more manipulable simply because they are less susceptible to peer and other review than are hospital visit lengths. Further research on this interpretation is needed before it can be viewed as anything more than speculative.

References

Berki, Sylvester, and Marie Ashcraft. 1980. "HMO enrollment: Who joins what and why: A review of the literature." *Milbank Memorial Fund Quarterly* 58:588–632.

Freidson, Eliot. 1970. *Profession of Medicine: A Study of the Sociology of Applied Knowledge.* New York: Harper and Row.

Freshnock, Larry, and Louis Goodman. 1980. "The organization of physician services in solo and group medical practice." *Medical Care* 18:17–29.

Hall, Oswald. 1946. "The informal organization of the medical profession." *Canadian Journal of Economics and Political Science* 12:30–41.

———. 1949. "Types of medical careers." *American Journal of Sociology* 55:243–53.

Held, Phillip, and Uwe Reinhardt. 1979. *Analysis of Economic Performance in Medical Group Practices.* Princeton: Mathematica Policy Research.

Kehrer, Barbara. 1976. "Factors affecting the incomes of men and women physicians: An exploratory study." *Journal of Human Resources* 11:526–39.

Krill, Mary, and Ralph Gaynor. 1982. "An assessment of the future of HMOs." *Medical Group Management* 29:42–46.

Langwell, Kathryn. 1982. "Factors affecting the incomes of men and women physicians: Further explorations." *Journal of Human Resources* 17:261–74.

Lewis-Beck, David. 1981. *Applied Regression Analysis.* Beverly Hills: Sage.

Luft, Harold. 1981. *Health Maintenance Organizations: Dimensions of Performance.* New York: Wiley.

———. 1983. "Health maintenance organizations." In *Handbook of Health, Health Care, and the Health Professions,* edited by David Mechanic. New York: Free Press.

Mechanic, David. 1975. "The organization of medical practice and practice orientations among physicians in prepaid and nonprepaid primary care settings." *Medical Care* 13:189–204.

———. 1979. "Correlates of physician utilization: Why do major multivariate studies of physician utilization find trivial psychosocial and organizational effects?" *Journal of Health and Social Behavior* 20:397–496.

Wolinsky, Fredric. 1980. "The performance of health maintenance organizations: An analytic review." *Milbank Memorial Fund Quarterly* 58:537–82.

———. 1982. "Why physicians choose different types of practice settings." *Health Services Research* 17:399–419.

Wolinsky, Fredric, and William Marder. 1982a. "HMOs: The concept, new evidence and implications." *Medical Group Management* 29:50–52, 58.

———. 1982b. "Spending time with patients: The impact of organizational structure on medical practice." *Medical Care* 20:1051–59.

———. 1983a. "Waiting to see the doctor: The impact of organizational structure on medical practice." *Medical Care* 21:531–42.

———. 1983b. "The organization of medical practice and primary care physician income." *American Journal of Public Health* 73:379–82.

4

The Organization of Medical Practice, Physician Workload Characteristics, Incomes, and Expenses

Overview

The purpose of this chapter is threefold. First, we describe the measures of physician workload characteristics, incomes, and expenses used to operationalize the general analytic model in assessing the effects of the organization of medical practice on the practice of medicine. Second, we use the general analytic model to focus on the effects of the organization of medical practice on physician workload characteristics. In particular, we examine two distinct aspects of physician workloads: (1) the total number of hours worked per week, as well as the number of direct patient care hours worked per week, and (2) the number of patients seen per week in the office and in the hospital. Finally, we use the general analytic model to study the effects of the organization of medical practice on physician incomes and expenses.

Operationalizing the Analytic Model for Physician Workload Characteristics, Incomes, and Expenses

The means, standard deviations, and coding algorithms of the variables used as measures of physician workload characteristics, incomes, and expenses are shown in table 4.1. The measures of the sociodemographic, environmental, and attitudinal characteristics are those described in chapter 3 and presented in table 3.1. As table 4.1 indicates, there are four measures of physician workload characteristics: the total number of hours worked per week, the number of direct patient care hours worked per week, the total number of patient visits per week in the office, and the total number of patient visits per week in the hospital. The first two of these measures are used to tap the global work effort of the physicians in our sample. Using the general analytic model to predict these two measures of physician workload characteristics allows us to assess whether or not the sociodemographic, environmental, attitudinal, and practice setting characteristics have a significant effect on the gross workload of physicians. In our sample, primary care physicians worked an average of 50.3 hours per week in their medical practice settings. Of this, an average of 45.3 hours per week were spent in direct patient care. As shown in the appendix, the total number of hours worked per week excludes "on call" hours not actually worked. Further, our measure of the number of direct patient care hours worked per week includes interpreting x-rays, lab tests, and the like, but excludes administrative tasks, meetings, and so forth.

The other two measures of physician workload characteristics shown in table 4.1 are the total number of patient visits per week, reported separately for the office and hospital. The primary care physicians in our sample reported an average of 96.7 patient visits per week in the office and an average of 28.5 patient visits per week in the hospital. Using the general analytic model to predict the effects of the sociodemographic, environmental, attitudinal, and practice setting characteristics on the total number of patient visits per week in the office and in the hospital allows us to focus more precisely on the distribution of hours practiced per week. If our theory is correct, we should observe statistically significant effects such that the regression coefficients for the practice setting characteristics demonstrate the distribution of patient visits between the office and the hospital to be affected by the practice setting. For example, if the extensive literature on the promise and performance of HMOs is accurate (Luft 1978a, 1978b, 1981, 1983; Wolinsky 1980), we would expect to find physicians practicing in HMOs (except those practicing in IPAs) to see more patients in the office and fewer in the hospital. This would support the argument that HMOs achieve their savings by providing more ambulatory as compared with institutional medical care.

Two measures of physician reimbursement are shown in table 4.1. The first is 1979 net individual income derived from medical practice. Primary care physicians report an average 1979 net individual income of $70,090 from medical practice. The second measure is total individual professional expenses in 1979. Primary care physicians report an average of $55,660 in expenses in 1979. Using the general analytic model to predict these two measures allows us to assess whether or not the sociodemographic, environmental, attitudinal, and practice setting characteristics have statistically significant effects on physician income and expenses. If, as Fink (1980) and others suggest, one of the difficulties of recruiting physicians into the various forms of HMOs is that HMO physicians are underpaid (relative to their fee-for-service counterparts), then we should find statistically significant negative regression coefficients for the HMO practice setting characteristics. Similarly, if Freidson (1970), Luft (1981), and others are correct

Table 4.1 Means, standard deviations, and coding algorithms of the variables in the general analytic model (*N* = 3,555)

Variables	Means	Standard Deviations	Coding Algorithms
Workload characteristics			
Total number of hours worked per week	50.317	13.405	Actual number of hours worked in most recent, complete week.
Number of direct patient care hours worked per week	45.321	14.285	Actual number of direct patient care hours worked in most recent, complete week.
Total number of patient visits per week: in the office	96.653	57.818	Actual number of patient office visits in most recent, complete week.
Total number of patient visits per week: in the hospital	28.475	32.904	Actual number of hospital visits in most recent, complete week.
Physician incomes and expenses			
Net 1979 individual income from medical practice	70.090	39.590	Thousands of dollars. (Natural logarithms used in the regression equations.)
Professional expenses in 1979	55.660	55.840	Thousands of dollars. (Natural logarithms used in the regression equations.)

in thinking that the more bureaucratic practice settings are attractive because professional expenses are more likely to be absorbed by the corporation, then we should find statistically significant negative coefficients for the more bureaucratic practice settings.

The Organization of Medical Practice and Physician Workload Characteristics

Tables 4.2 and 4.3 show the regression coefficients, intercepts, and squared multiple correlation coefficients (R^2) obtained from the hierarchical modeling process to evaluate the general analytic model in assessing the total number of hours and the number of direct patient care hours worked per week. At the most general level, a comparison of the R^2 coefficients for models 1, 2, and 3 indicates no support for the general analytic model. Focusing first on modeling the total number of hours worked per week (table 4.2), model 1 (i.e., the sociodemographic and environmental characteristics) explains 10.4 percent of the variance in the total number of hours worked per week. When the attitudinal characteristics are added into the equation in model 2, the explained variance rises, but only to 11.1 percent. This modest increase in explanatory power is consistent with the emergence of a few statistically significant effects for the attitudinal measures which we shall discuss shortly. Most important for our theory, however, is the failure of the introduction of the practice setting characteristics in model 3 to increase the explanatory power. Indeed, the explained variance in model 3 increases only 0.2 percent, to 11.3 percent. This miniscule increase indicates the absence of any statistically significant effect for the practice setting characteristics on the number of hours worked per week.

When the hierarchical modeling procedure is used to predict the number of direct patient care hours worked per week, we observe the same pattern. The R^2 coefficients shown in table 4.3 indicate that when the sociodemographic and environmental characteristics are used to predict the number of direct patient care hours worked per week in model 1, 9.0 percent of the variance is explained. When the attitudinal characteristics are introduced in model 2, the explained variance rises only to 9.4 percent, as reflected by the fact that only one of the attitudinal characteristics produced a statistically significant effect. Most important for our theory, however, is the fact that when the practice setting characteristics are added into the equation in model 3, the explained variance rises only to 9.5 percent. None of the practice setting characteristics produce statistically significant effects on the number of direct patient care hours worked per week.

Overall, then, the comparisons of the R^2 coefficients for models 1, 2, and 3 indicate three things. First, the sociodemographic and environmental characteristics account for most of the explained variance obtained in modeling the total number of hours and the number of direct patient care hours worked per week. Second, the inclusion of the attitudinal characteristics in model 2 adds less than 1.0 percent to the explained variance. Third, the inclusion of the practice setting characteristics in model 3 adds no more than 0.2 percent to the explanatory power of the general analytic model.

We now focus on the effects of the sociodemographic, environmental, attitudinal, and practice setting characteristics reflected in the regression coefficients obtained in models 1, 2, and 3. Table 4.2 reveals that all of the sociodemographic characteristics, except the dummy variable for pediatrics, have a statistically significant effect on the total number of hours worked per week. Moreover, the subsequent introduction of the attitudinal and practice setting characteristics in models

Table 4.2 Partial regression and R^2 coefficients, T-ratios, and probability levels obtained from the hierarchical modeling of the total number of hours worked per week

Variables	Model 1 b	Model 1 T-Ratio	Model 1 Probability Level	Model 2 b	Model 2 T-Ratio	Model 2 Probability Level	Model 3 b	Model 3 T-Ratio	Model 3 Probability Level
Sociodemographic characteristics									
Sex	-6.561	-6.92	.000	-6.376	-6.74	.000	-6.289	-6.64	.000
AMA membership	3.758	8.00	.000	3.654	7.78	.000	3.542	7.45	.000
Board certified	2.443	5.09	.000	2.472	5.14	.000	2.490	5.09	.000
Experience	-0.237	-12.09	.000	-0.236	-11.97	.000	-0.238	-11.86	.000
Internal medicine	2.833	5.24	.000	2.855	5.29	.000	2.938	5.42	.000
Pediatrics	-0.400	-0.56	.574	-0.348	-0.49	.624	-0.197	-0.28	.783
OB/GYN	1.407	2.01	.045	1.513	2.16	.031	1.605	2.29	.022
Environmental characteristics									
Western U.S.	-1.310	-2.51	.012	-1.376	-2.63	.009	-1.111	-2.01	.045
MD/POP ratio	-1.253	-0.91	.363	-1.237	-0.90	.368	-0.975	-0.71	.480
Local income	-0.815	-2.97	.003	-0.768	-2.80	.005	-0.722	-2.62	.009
Local education	-2.282	-0.69	.489	-0.326	-0.80	.422	-0.350	-0.86	.389
Attitudinal characteristics									
Business side				1.457	2.64	.008	1.500	2.70	.007
Scheduling ease				-1.742	-3.49	.001	-1.671	-3.32	.001
Personal autonomy				1.010	2.22	.026	0.853	1.77	.077
Practice location				0.976	1.99	.47	1.015	2.07	.039
Earnings potential				-0.305	-0.46	.648	-0.380	-0.57	.569
Practice setting characteristics									
Kaiser HMO							-1.811	-1.32	.187
Non-Kaiser group HMO							-2.497	-1.91	.056
Staff HMO							-1.918	-1.37	.172
Staff HMO							-0.341	-0.57	.566
Solo F-F-S							-0.000	-0.00	.999
Intercept	59.237	36.12	.000	.870	26.52	.000	59.140	20.52	.000
R^2	.104	36.12	.000	.111			.113		

Table 4.3 Partial regression and R^2 coefficients, *T*-ratios, and probability levels obtained from the hierarchical modeling of the number of direct patient care hours worked per week

Variables	Model 1 b	Model 1 T-Ratio	Model 1 Probability Level	Model 2 b	Model 2 T-Ratio	Model 2 Probability Level	Model 3 b	Model 3 T-Ratio	Model 3 Probability Level
Sociodemographic characteristics									
Sex	-6.538	-6.45	.000	-6.417	-6.33	.000	-6.348	-6.26	.000
AMA membership	4.275	8.51	.000	4.204	8.37	.000	4.133	8.12	.000
Board certified	1.609	3.13	.002	1.649	3.20	.001	1.663	3.17	.002
Experience	-0.229	-11.03	.000	-0.227	-10.85	.000	-0.229	-10.73	.000
Internal medicine	2.263	3.91	.000	2.280	3.94	.000	2.342	4.03	.000
Pediatrics	-0.393	-0.51	.607	-0.344	-0.45	.652	-0.244	-0.32	.751
OB/GYN	1.720	2.28	.023	1.759	2.33	.020	1.821	2.41	.016
Environmental characteristics									
Western U.S.	0.734	-1.31	.191	-0.789	-1.40	.161	-0.626	-1.05	.293
MD/POP ratio	-4.649	-3.13	.002	-4.681	-3.15	.002	-4.349	-2.91	.004
Local income	-1.153	-3.93	.000	-1.111	-3.78	.000	-1.080	-3.66	.000
Local education	0.101	0.23	.816	0.061	0.14	.889	0.047	0.11	.915
Attitudinal characteristics									
Business side				1.115	1.88	.061	1.145	1.92	.055
Scheduling ease				-1.078	-2.01	.044	-1.049	-1.94	.053
Personal autonomy				0.931	1.91	.057	0.857	1.65	.098
Practice location				0.846	1.61	.107	0.864	1.64	.101
Earnings potential				-0.268	-0.37	.709	-0.339	-0.47	.636
Practice setting characteristics									
Kaiser HMO							-0.572	-0.39	.700
Non-Kaiser group HMO							-2.685	-1.92	.055
Staff HMO							-2.315	-1.53	.127
IPA HMO							-0.389	-0.61	.541
Solo F-F-S							-0.148	-0.27	.785
Intercept	52.265			51.806			52.054		
R^2	.090	30.87	.000	.094	22.10	.000	.095	17.11	.000

2 and 3 do not alter in any meaningful way the effects of the sociodemographic characteristics obtained from model 1. Basically, the effects of the sociodemographic characteristics are as follows. Female physicians work about 6.3 fewer total hours per week than their male counterparts. Physicians who are members of the AMA work about 3.5 more hours per week than non-AMA members. Board certified physicians work about 2.5 more hours per week than do non-board certified physicians. With each additional year of experience, physicians work about a quarter of an hour less per week.

The effects of the dummy variables for medical specialty indicate the following. Internists have the longest work weeks, spending about 2.9 hours more per week than their family or general practitioner counterparts. Obstetrician/gynecologists have the next longest work week, spending about 1.6 more hours per week than general or family practitioners. Pediatricians do not work any more or fewer hours than general or family practice physicians. These specialty differences may, in part, explain why internists and obstetrician/gynecologists have significantly higher incomes than their pediatrics and family or general practice counterparts: they work significantly longer hours per week.

For the environmental characteristics, we find that the effects obtained in model 1 are also unaltered when the attitudinal characteristics are introduced in model 2, and when the practice setting characteristics are introduced in model 3. That is, the effect (or lack of an effect) of the environmental characteristics is neither spurious to nor suppressed by the attitudinal and practice setting characteristics. The western United States variable produces a statistically significant negative effect. On average, physicians who practice in the western United States work about 1.1 fewer hours per week than those in other regions. The physician-to-population ratio appears to be unrelated to the total number of hours worked per week. Mean local income produces a statistically significant negative effect on the total number of hours worked per week. This regression coefficient indicates that for each $1,000 increase in average areal income, we should see a concomitant 0.7 hour decrease in the total number of hours worked per week by physicians. Finally, the local median educational level appears to be unrelated to the total number of hours worked per week by physicians.

The effects of the attitudinal characteristics on the total number of hours worked per week are positive for the business side of practice, personal autonomy, and practice location, and negative for scheduling ease. Physicians who consider the business side of medical practice to be very important in selecting a practice setting work about 1.5 more hours per week than their counterparts who view it as less important. Physicians who consider personal autonomy to be very important in the selection of a practice setting work about 1.0 more hours per week than their counterparts who feel otherwise. When the practice setting characteristics are introduced in model 3, however, the positive effect of personal autonomy is diminished to insignificance. Physicians who consider practice location to be very important work about 1.0 more hours per week. Finally, physicians who consider scheduling ease to be very important in selecting a new practice work about 1.7 fewer hours per week.

It is intuitively pleasing to find that physicians who work longer hours are those who consider the business side of practice and personal autonomy to be salient issues in selecting a new practice setting; we would expect business-oriented individuals to work longer hours. Similarly, it is also understandable that physicians who consider scheduling ease to be very important in selecting a new practice work fewer hours per week; these physicians appear to concentrate on efficiency. The significant effect of practice location is somewhat less straightforward, but we will not address it here. What appears counterintuitive, however, is the absence of a statistically significant effect for earnings potential. That is, one would assume that physicians who value earnings potential in the selection of a practice setting would be more likely to work longer hours per week. The absence of a statistically significant effect for earnings potential may, however, indicate that physicians holding these attitudes use non-labor intensive activities to generate greater earnings. Unfortunately, this issue cannot be explored further with these data.

Turning to the effects of the practice setting characteristics, the results provide no support for our theory. That is, none of the practice setting characteristics produced a statistically significant effect on the total number of hours that physicians work per week. Indeed, the only effect that approaches statistical significance is for physicians in non-Kaiser group model HMOs, who work fewer, but not statistically significantly fewer, hours per week than their counterparts in group fee-for-service practices. Although these data do not support our theory, they may not completely refute it either. While the organization of medical practice may not be related to this gross measure of physician workload (the total number of hours worked per week), it may affect the distribution of work within the "normal" work week (for example, how hours are distributed between the office and the hospital). Further analysis of the workload characteristics will bear more directly on this issue.

The results obtained from models 1, 2, and 3 in predicting the number of direct patient care hours are very similar to those obtained for the total number of hours worked per week. At the general level, the R^2 coefficients obtained from modeling the number of direct patient care hours worked per week are very similar, for all three models, to those obtained for the total number of hours worked per week. The effects of the four sets of characteristics (sociodemographic, environmental, attitudinal, and practice setting) obtained from modeling the number of direct patient care hours worked per week are also similar to those obtained from modeling the total number of hours worked per week, although there are some differences. We shall concentrate on those differences.

Among the sociodemographic characteristics, the dummy variable for pediatrics is again the only measure that does not produce a statistically significant effect on the number of direct patient care hours worked per week. Female physicians have about 6.3 fewer hours of direct patient care per week than their male counterparts. Members of the AMA have about 4.1 more hours and board certified physicians about 1.7 more hours of direct patient care than do their opposite numbers. Experience produced approximately the same negative effect on the number of direct patient care hours that it did for the total number of hours worked per week; with each additional year of experience, physicians work about two-tenths of an hour less per week.

Turning to the effects of the set of dummy variables measuring medical specialty, we find that internists again have the greatest number of direct patient care hours, averaging 2.3 more hours than their family or general practice counterparts. Obstetrician/gynecologists have the next largest number of direct patient care hours, averaging about 1.8 more hours per week than their family or general practice counterparts. Again, pediatricians do not have significantly more or fewer direct patient care hours per week than their general or family practice counterparts.

At this point it is important to note that the effects of all of the sociodemographic characteristics obtained in model 1 remain virtually the same in models 2 and 3. Thus, as was the case with number of hours worked per week, the effects of the sociodemographic characteristics on the number of direct patient care hours per week are virtually unaltered by the introduction of either the attitudinal or the practice setting characteristics.

As indicated in table 4.3, the effects of the environmental characteristics are slightly different for direct patient care hours and total number of hours worked per week. In predicting the number of direct patient care hours worked per week, it is the physician-to-population ratio and the local average income that produce statistically significant effects. The western United States and local median educational level variables are unrelated to the number of patient care hours worked per week. The effect of the physician-to-population ratio is negative, indicating that the larger the supply of physicians relative to the population, the fewer the hours of direct patient care. This is expected, and indicates that where competition is greater, physicians average fewer hours of direct patient care. The effect of local average income level is also negative, as it was for the total number of hours worked per week. This statistically significant negative effect may indicate that in more affluent areal markets there is less need for medical care, especially restorative care, which can require more lengthy patient contact. Thus, physicians can "get by" with fewer hours per week for direct patient care. Finally, it is again worth noting that the effects of the environmental characteristics obtained from model 1 are virtually unaffected by the introduction of the attitudinal and practice setting characteristics introduced in models 2 and 3. That is, the effects of the environmental characteristics are also neither spurious to nor suppressed by the attitudinal and practice setting characteristics.

When the attitudinal characteristics are introduced in model 2, only the scheduling ease variable produces a statistically significant effect on the number of direct patient care hours worked per week. This effect is again negative, indicating that physicians who view scheduling ease as very important in selecting a practice setting have about 1.1 fewer hours of direct patient care per week than their counterparts. None of the other attitudinal characteristics introduced in model 2 produce statistically significant effects. Moreover, when the practice setting characteristics are introduced in model 3, the statistically significant effect of scheduling ease is reduced to insignificance. Thus, the results presented in table 4.3 indicate that the attitudinal characteristics have no statistically significant effect on the number of direct patient care hours worked per week, net of the effects of the sociodemographic, environmental, and practice setting characteristics.

As for the practice setting characteristics introduced in model 3, the pattern for the number of direct patient care hours worked per week is the same as for the total number of hours worked per week. Once again, none of the coefficients for the set of dummy variables measuring the practice settings is statistically significant. Indeed, the only practice setting characteristic that even approaches statistical significance is the effect of being in a non-Kaiser group model HMO. This coefficient indicates that physicians in non-Kaiser group model HMOs spend fewer hours in direct patient care than their group fee-for-service counterparts, the same non-effect that we found concerning the total number of hours worked per week. Thus, the results obtained for the practice setting characteristics reported in table 4.3 also fail to provide any support for our theory.

However, as suggested in reviewing the absence of support for our theory in table 4.2, the data reported in table 4.3 do not rule out the possibility of a relationship between the organization of medical practice and physician workload characteristics. The data presented in tables 4.2 and 4.3 clearly show that the average number of hours worked per week or spent in direct patient care is unrelated to the organization of medical practice. It is, however, still possible that the distribution of hours between the office and hospital settings within the average physician's work week is so related. Accordingly, we now turn to the application of the general analytic model to the number of office and hospital visits that occur per week.

Tables 4.4 and 4.5 contain the regression coefficients, intercepts, and R^2 coefficients obtained from the hierarchical modeling of the number of office visits and hospital visits per week. At the most general level, comparing the R^2 coefficients for models 1, 2, and 3 in tables 4.4 and 4.5, we do not find much support for the general analytic model. The sociodemographic and environmental characteristics contained in model 1 are able to explain 20.5 percent of the variance in the number of office visits per week and 12.4 percent of the variance in the number of hospital visits per week. When the attitudinal characteristics are added in model 2, the explained variance for the number of office visits remains unchanged, and the explained variance for the number of hospital visits increases by only 0.1 percent. Thus, the introduction of the attitudinal characteristics in model 2 does not significantly contribute to the prediction of either office or hospital visits (although the business side of medical practice variable produces a statistically significant effect on the number of office visits). Similarly, the introduction of the practice setting characteristics in model 3 increases the explained variance for the number of office visits to only 21.5 percent, a 1.0 percent increment. The introduction of the practice setting characteristics in model 3 increases the explained variance of the number of hospital visits to only 13.3 percent, a 0.8 percent increment. Thus, it appears that the practice setting characteristics are basically unrelated to the number of office and hospital visits.

Several of the practice setting characteristics, however, produced statistically significant effects on the number of office encounters per week and on the number of hospital visits per week. Because no major increment in explained variance is achieved by the introduction of the practice setting characteristics, these data indicate that a significant portion of the effects of the sociodemographic and environmental characteristics in models 1 and 2 was spuriously associated with those characteristics. The introduction of the practice setting characteristics in model 3 allows these effects to be properly credited to the organization of medical practice. Therefore, in the more focused examination of the effects of the sociodemographic and environmental characteristics that follows, we should be able to identify the relationships that are diminished by the introduction of the practice setting characteristics.

We now turn our attention to the effects on the number of office visits by the sociodemographic, environmental, attitudinal, and practice setting characteristics, indicated by the regression coefficients in models 1, 2, and 3 (see table 4.4). Beginning with the sociodemographic characteristics, we see that female physicians average about 20 fewer office visits per week than their male counterparts. This gender gap remains relatively constant across all three models. Physicians who are members of the AMA have an average of 10 more office visits per week than their non-AMA counterparts; this relationship is also relatively constant across all three models. Board certified physicians average about 4.8 more office visits per week than non-board certified physicians, at least according to the results obtained for models 1 and 2. When the practice setting characteristics are introduced in model 3, however, the differential in office visits per week between board certified and non-board certified physicians declines to an average of 4.4. More experienced physicians have fewer office visits per week, averaging about .39 fewer visits per week for each additional year of experience that they

Table 4.4 Partial regression and R^2 coefficients, T-ratios, and probability levels obtained from the hierarchical modeling of the number of office visits per week

Variables	Model 1			Model 2			Model 3		
	b	T-Ratio	Probability Level	b	T-Ratio	Probability Level	b	T-Ratio	Probability Level
Sociodemographic characteristics									
Sex	-19.841	-5.10	.000	-19.631	-5.05	.000	-19.962	-5.14	.000
AMA membership	10.019	5.25	.000	9.804	5.14	.000	10.248	5.33	.000
Board certified	4.829	2.47	.014	4.803	2.45	.014	4.373	2.20	.028
Experience	-0.394	-5.00	.000	-0.360	-4.54	.000	-0.343	-4.25	.000
Internal medicine	-45.057	-20.51	.000	-44.779	-20.41	.000	-45.474	-20.70	.000
Pediatrics	9.640	3.33	.001	9.380	3.25	.001	7.990	2.75	.006
OB/GYN	-17.634	-6.19	.000	-17.898	-6.28	.000	-18.388	-6.46	.000
Environmental characteristics									
Western U.S.	0.853	0.40	.688	0.796	0.37	.709	-1.630	-0.73	.468
MD/POP ratio	-38.027	-6.88	.000	-38.235	-6.92	.000	-38.399	-6.93	.000
Local income	-0.401	-0.36	.719	-0.397	-0.36	.722	-0.463	-0.42	.678
Local education	-8.091	-4.88	.000	-8.030	-4.84	.000	-8.126	-4.91	.000
Attitudinal characteristics									
Business side				5.270	2.35	.091	4.982	2.23	.026
Scheduling ease				0.385	0.19	.849	-0.489	-0.24	.810
Personal autonomy				-2.197	-1.19	.234	-0.553	-0.28	.778
Practice location				0.302	0.15	.879	0.269	0.14	.892
Earnings potential				5.177	1.91	.057	5.224	1.93	.054
Practice setting characteristics									
Kaiser HMO							22.245	3.98	.000
Non-Kaiser group HMO							7.831	1.47	.141
Staff HMO							-12.632	-2.22	.026
IPA HMO							2.660	1.11	.269
Solo F-F-S							2.998	-1.46	.145
Intercept	223.027			220.464			222.562		
R^2	.205	80.08	.000	.205	80.08	.000	.215	44.50	.000

Table 4.5 Partial regression and R^2 coefficients, *T*-ratios, and probability levels obtained from the hierarchical modeling of the number of hospital visits per week

Variables	Model 1			Model 2			Model 3		
	b	T-Ratio	Probability Level	b	T-Ratio	Probability Level	b	T-Ratio	Probability Level
Sociodemographic characteristics									
Sex	-6.217	-2.52	.012	-6.023	-2.44	.015	-5.713	-2.32	.020
AMA membership	7.730	6.69	.000	7.646	6.60	.000	7.048	6.04	.000
Board certified	4.136	3.50	.001	4.144	3.49	.001	3.390	2.82	.005
Experience	-0.281	-5.86	.000	-0.287	-5.92	.000	-0.255	-5.18	.000
Internal medicine	13.223	9.95	.000	13.247	9.97	.000	13.213	9.93	.000
Pediatrics	-6.044	-3.45	.001	-6.136	-3.50	.001	-6.330	-3.59	.000
OB/GYN	-2.390	-1.39	.166	-2.231	-1.29	.197	-2.300	-1.33	.183
Environmental characteristics									
Western U.S.	-10.259	-7.96	.000	-10.219	-7.91	.000	-9.577	-7.02	.000
MD/POP ratio	-13.844	-4.08	.000	-13.792	-4.06	.000	-12.775	-3.75	.000
Local income	-0.311	-0.46	.644	-0.286	-0.42	.671	-0.133	-0.20	.844
Local education	-3.870	-3.85	.000	-3.886	-3.86	.000	-3.940	-3.92	.000
Attitudinal characteristics									
Business side				1.061	0.78	.436	0.959	0.71	.481
Scheduling ease				-1.811	-1.47	.140	-2.073	-1.68	.093
Personal autonomy				-1.024	-0.91	.361	-0.073	-0.06	.951
Practice location				-1.301	-1.08	.281	-1.254	-1.04	.298
Earnings potential				0.631	0.38	.703	0.418	0.25	.800
Practice setting characteristics									
Kaiser HMO							-7.810	-2.29	.022
Non-Kaiser group HMO							-12.444	3.74	.000
Staff HMO							-4.448	-1.29	.198
IPA HMO							-1.061	-0.73	.466
Solo F-F-S							-5.110	-4.12	.000
Intercept	78.066	42.76	.000	79.531	29.73	.000	81.973	24.30	.000
R^2	.124			.125			.133		

accrue. Like the board certification effect, though, the experience effect is also slightly diminished when the practice setting characteristics are introduced in model 3.

Clearly the largest effects of the sociodemographic characteristics on the number of office visits per week are obtained for the set of dummy variables measuring medical specialty. Internists have the fewest office visits per week, obstetrician/gynecologists the next fewest, followed by general or family practitioners. Pediatricians have the largest number of office visits per week. Internists have about 45.5 fewer office visits per week than their general or family practice counterparts, and this differential is unaffected by the introduction of the practice setting characteristics. Obstetrician/gynecologists have about 18.4 fewer office visits per week than their family or general practice counterparts, and this differential is also unaffected by the introduction of the practice setting characteristics in model 3. Pediatricians, on the other hand, have about 8.0 more office visits per week than their general or family practice counterparts. The pediatrics differential, however, is reduced by about 1.4 visits per week with the introduction of the practice setting characteristics in model 3.

Among the environmental characteristics, there are three interesting points to note. First, the western United States and local income variables never produce statistically significant effects on the number of office visits per week. This indicates that the average number of office visits worked per week on the west coast is no different from that in the other regions of the country, and that the number of office visits worked per week is not related to local income levels. Second, the physician-to-population ratio produces a significant negative effect on the number of office visits worked per week, and this effect is not altered by the introduction of either the attitudinal or the practice setting characteristics. The negative effect of the physician-to-population ratio on the number of office visits per week indicates that the greater the competition among physicians for patients, the fewer office visits each will have. Moreover, these regression coefficients indicate that for every increase of one physician per 100 county inhabitants, each physician would have about 38.4 fewer office visits. Although an increase in the physician-to-population ratio of one per 100 is unlikely, an increase of one per 1,000 is not at all unlikely, and would result in approximately 4.0 fewer office visits per physician per week. Thus, these data suggest that the number of office visits is not inelastic with regard to the physician-to-population ratio.

The third interesting point to note from the effects of the environmental characteristics shown in table 4.4 is the significant negative effect of local median educational levels on the number of office visits. On average, a one-year increment in the local median educational level would result in 8.1 fewer office visits per week per physician. This probably reflects the fact that health status levels are higher in areas where local educational levels are also higher, and thus there is less need (i.e., demand) for physicians' services. Like the negative effect of the physician-to-population ratio, the negative effect of the local median educational level remains relatively constant across all three models.

The effect of the attitudinal characteristics on the number of office visits per week is minimal and is principally limited to the significant positive effect of the business side of medical practice. Physicians who report that the business of medicine was an important issue in selecting a practice setting have about 5.3 more office visits per week than other physicians. This effect is basically unaltered by the introduction of the practice setting characteristics in model 3. The only other attitudinal characteristic that produces an effect even approaching statistical significance is the importance of earnings potential in the selection of a medical practice. Although not quite statistically significant, physicians who consider earnings potential to be very important have about 5.0 more office visits per week. The statistically significant effect of the business side of practice and the nearly statistically significant effect of earnings potential on the number of office visits per week are intuitive and straightforward. That is, we would expect physicians who are more concerned with business and with earnings potential to have more office visits.

The data in table 4.4 on the effects of the practice setting characteristics provide considerable support for our theory, although this support may not seem quite clear until we have discussed the results reported in table 4.5. Only two of the practice setting characteristics produce statistically significant effects on the number of office visits. Physicians in Kaiser model HMOs have about 22.2 *more* office visits per week than their counterparts in group fee-for-service. This is as we would expect, given that Luft (1981, 1983) and others (Wolinsky 1980) have argued that the way in which HMOs achieve their cost savings is by substituting ambulatory or office visits for hospital visits.

What is not consistent with our theory, however, is the absence of a statistically significant effect of the non-Kaiser group model HMO variable, and the presence of a statistically significant negative effect for the staff model HMO variable. Although not statistically significant, the effect of the non-Kaiser group model HMO variable is positive, suggesting that there is a tendency for physicians in this practice setting to have more office visits than their group fee-for-service counterparts. This is as we would expect, although we had expected this effect to be strong enough to be statistically significant. The statistically significant negative effect of the staff model HMO variable, however, is counter-intuitive. That is, like physicians in Kaiser and non-Kaiser group model HMOs (although not as much like them), we expected physicians in staff model HMOs to provide more office visits coupled with fewer hospital visits per week. This is not the case. We shall delay further discussion of this apparently aberrant finding until we review the effects of the practice setting characteristics on the number of hospital visits per week shown in table 4.5.

The effects of the two remaining practice setting characteristics are basically as we expected. Physicians in IPA model HMOs do not have significantly more or fewer office visits per week than their counterparts in group fee-for-service practice. This is intuitively pleasing, since we have argued all along that IPA model HMO physicians face the same incentive and reimbursement structures as those in group fee-for-service. Similarly, physicians in solo fee-for-service practice do not have significantly more or fewer office visits per week than group fee-for-service physicians. We expected this, as well, because the reimbursement incentives in these two practice settings are the same.

Table 4.5 contains the results of the hierarchical modeling of the number of hospital visits per week. Among the effects of the sociodemographic characteristics we find that female physicians have about 6.2 fewer hospital visits per week than male physicians. However, with the introduction of the attitudinal and practice setting characteristics in models 2 and 3, this gender differential is reduced to about 5.7 hospital visits per week. Coupled with the gender differences obtained from modeling the number of office visits per week, these data indicate that female physicians see significantly fewer patients per week, both in the office and in the hospital.

Physicians who are members of the AMA have about 7.7 more hospital visits per week than do their non-AMA member counterparts. When the practice setting characteristics are introduced in model 3, this AMA membership differential is reduced, falling to about 7.0 visits per week. Board certified physicians also have more hospital visits per week than do their non-board certified counterparts; here the difference is about 4.1 visits per week. Again, however, when the practice setting characteristics are introduced in model 3, this board certification differential is reduced to about 3.4 hospital visits per week. When combined with the data on the number of office visits per week, the data shown in table 4.5 indicate that members of the AMA and board certified physicians have significantly more office and hospital visits per week. Similarly, the effect of experience on the number of hospital visits per week is much as it was on the number of office visits. For every additional year of experience physicians accrue, they are likely to reduce hospital visits by about one-fourth of a visit per week.

The effects of the set of dummy variables for medical specialty reveal several interesting results. First, while internists had the fewest office visits per week, they have the most hospital visits, averaging about 13.2 more visits per week than their general or family practice counterparts. Similarly, while pediatricians had the greatest number of office visits per week, they have the fewest hospital visits, averaging about 6.3 fewer visits per week than general or family practice physicians. Obstetrician/gynecologists and general or family practitioners fall between these two extremes, the obstetrician/gynecologists having slightly fewer (but not significantly fewer) hospital visits. Thus, the effects of the medical specialty dummy variables shown in tables 4.4 and 4.5 indicate that the practice of some medical specialties is more concentrated in the office, others more in hospitals.

Moreover, there appears to be an offsetting distribution of visits between the two settings across the medical specialties.

Turning to the environmental characteristics, we note four interesting points. First, local income levels are not significantly related to the number of hospital visits per week. Indeed, the regression coefficients for local income do not even approach statistical significance in any of the three models. Second, the western United States variable has a statistically significant negative effect on the number of hospital visits per week, with physicians in the western United States making about 10.3 fewer hospital visits per week than physicians in other geographic regions. When the practice setting characteristics are introduced in model 3, however, this geographic differential is reduced to about 9.6 hospital visits per week. When coupled with the results obtained from modeling the number of office visits per week, these data indicate that although physicians in the western United States may hospitalize fewer patients (i.e., they have fewer hospital visits per week), they do not compensate for the associated loss of patient visits by increasing the number of office visits per week.

The third and fourth interesting effects of the environmental characteristics are similar to those observed for the number of office visits per week. Higher physician-to-population ratios result in significantly fewer hospital visits. Moreover, this differential is only slightly diminished by the introduction of the practice setting characteristics in model 3. An increase in the physician supply on the order of one physician for every 1,000 persons in the county would result in about 1.3 fewer hospital visits per physician per week. Again, this is intuitively straightforward, indicating that the number of hospital visits per physician is not unrelated to the supply of (i.e., competition among) physicians.

Likewise, the effect of local median educational levels on the number of hospital visits per week is also significantly negative, as it was for office visits. Moreover, the introduction of the attitudinal and practice setting characteristics in models 2 and 3 does not alter this basic effect. The effect is such that if the median educational level is increased by one year of formal schooling, the number of hospital visits per physician per week would decrease by about 3.9. Again, this probably reflects the fact that higher educational levels are associated with healthier patient populations, and thus there is less need (i.e., demand) for physicians' services.

The introduction of the attitudinal characteristics in models 2 and 3 results in a very straightforward pattern of effects (or actually noneffects). None of the attitudinal characteristics produced statistically significant effects on the number of hospital visits per week in either models 2 or 3. Although we had expected some significant relationships would emerge between the attitudinal characteristics and the number of hospital visits, the absence of these relationships is not necessarily counter-intuitive. That is, the attitudinal characteristics consist of five issues that physicians reported were either very important or not very important in their selection of a practice setting. Because these practice setting issues relate primarily to the office, it is not surprising that they do not significantly affect the number of hospital visits.

Turning to the effects of the practice setting characteristics, we again find considerable support for our theory. This support becomes more obvious when we consider the effects of the practice setting characteristics shown in table 4.5 in conjunction with those shown in table 4.4. In table 4.5 significant negative effects are found for the Kaiser model HMO and the non-Kaiser group model HMO variables. Physicians in Kaiser model HMOs have about 7.8 fewer, and physicians in non-Kaiser group model HMOs have about 12.4 fewer hospital visits per week than their group fee-for-service counterparts. When coupled with the fact that physicians in these two practice settings also had significantly more (almost so for non-Kaiser group model HMOs) office visits per week, their significantly fewer hospital visits per week suggest that these physicians are substituting ambulatory care for hospital-based care. The results for physicians in staff model HMOs do not support our theory, however. They have fewer hospital visits than their group fee-for-service counterparts, but not significantly fewer. That physicians in IPA model HMOs have no more or fewer hospital visits than those in group fee-for-service is also consistent with our theoretical expectations. Again, we expect this noneffect because these IPA model HMO physicians face the same reimbursement and incentive structures as in group fee-for-service.

The significant negative effect of the solo fee-for-service variable shown in table 4.5 appears to be somewhat anomalous. This effect indicates that physicians in solo fee-for-service make about 5.1 fewer hospital visits per week than their group fee-for-service counterparts. Given that they have the same reimbursement incentives (i.e., fee-for-service), we would not have expected them to have either significantly more or fewer hospital visits. However, further reflection on the special circumstances of the solo practice physician may explain this finding. It may be that solo practice physicians have significantly fewer hospital visits because of the coverage problems created when they leave their office settings to make their hospital rounds. Group fee-for-service practice physicians may easily arrange coverage among their on-site partners; solo practitioners must either arrange for coverage at another site or spend far more time traveling back and forth between the hospital and the office. As a result, solo practitioners may simply be constrained from providing as many hospital visits as their group fee-for-service counterparts.

Although tables 4.2, 4.3, 4.4, and 4.5 present the precise effects on the total number of hours worked per week, the number of patient care hours worked per week, and the number of office and hospital visits per week, they do not intuitively portray the magnitude of the differences in these workload characteristics across the various organizational forms of medical practice. To compensate for these shortcomings, we have again used the precise effects of the general analytic model to adjust these workload characteristics within each of the six practice settings for differences in the sociodemographic, environmental, and attitudinal characteristics. Table 4.6 shows the results of these calculations, which basically adjust the practice setting means by removing the differences due to the socio-demographic, environmental, and attitudinal characteristics. As the adjusted means in table 4.6 indicate, there are virtually no meaningful differences across the six practice settings on the total number of hours worked per week or on the number of direct patient care hours worked per week. There are, however, meaningful differences in the number of office and hospital visits per week, and these differences are generally consistent with our theoretical expectations. Thus, the data in table 4.6 flesh out a more intuitively pleasing demonstration of the support for our theory among the office and hospital visit measures than can be obtained solely from the hierarchical regression results presented in tables 4.4 and 4.5.

The Organization of Medical Practice, Physician Incomes, and Expenses

Tables 4.7 and 4.8 contain the regression coefficients, intercepts, and R^2 coefficients obtained from using the general analytic model to predict net individual physician incomes and expenses from medical practice. At this point, we remind the reader that although table 4.1 contains the means and standard deviations in thousands of dollars for net incomes and expenses, the hierarchical regression models reported in tables 4.7 and 4.8 refer to the natural logarithms of those dollars.

Table 4.6   Average adjusted means for the workload characteristics by practice setting

	Average Adjusted Workload Characteristic Mean			
Practice Setting	*Total Hours Worked*	*Patient Care Hours*	*Number of Office Visits*	*Number of Hospital Visits*
Kaiser model HMO	48.7	45.1	120.0	23.6
Non-Kaiser group model HMO	48.0	43.3	105.7	18.9
Staff model HMO	48.6	43.3	85.2	26.9
IPA model HMO	50.2	45.3	100.5	30.3
Group F-F-S	50.5	45.6	97.8	31.4
Solo F-F-S	50.5	45.5	94.8	26.3

Note: Means are adjusted for differences in the sociodemographic, environmental, and attitudinal characteristics used in the general analytic model.

Table 4.7 Partial regression and R^2 coefficients, *T*-ratios, and probability levels obtained from the hierarchical modeling of net 1979 individual income from medical practice

Variables	Model 1 b	Model 1 T-Ratio	Model 1 Probability Level	Model 2 b	Model 2 T-Ratio	Model 2 Probability Level	Model 3 b	Model 3 T-Ratio	Model 3 Probability Level
Sociodemographic characteristics									
Sex	−0.431	−11.08	.000	−0.426	−10.98	.000	−0.426	−10.99	.000
AMA membership	0.164	8.53	.000	0.160	8.39	.000	0.162	8.37	.000
Board certified	0.120	6.03	.000	0.123	6.19	.000	0.121	6.00	.000
Experience	0.046	15.76	.000	0.047	15.96	.000	0.047	15.83	.000
Experience^2	−0.001	−17.87	.000	−0.001	−17.98	.000	−0.001	−17.90	.000
Internal medicine	0.168	7.59	.000	0.171	7.73	.000	0.170	7.68	.000
Pediatrics	−0.005	−0.18	.855	−0.006	−0.22	.829	−0.009	−0.29	.769
OB/GYN	0.325	11.29	.000	0.322	11.21	.000	0.321	11.20	.000
Environmental characteristics									
Western U.S.	−0.005	−0.24	.809	−0.001	−0.04	.969	−0.006	−0.25	.805
MD/POP ratio	−0.128	−2.38	.017	−0.123	−2.30	.022	−0.108	−2.01	.045
Local income	0.016	1.41	.160	0.013	1.14	.255	0.014	1.25	.211
Local education	−0.054	−3.22	.001	−0.051	3.04	.002	−0.052	−3.10	.002
Attitudinal characteristics									
Business side				0.030	1.31	.189	0.028	1.26	.206
Scheduling ease				−0.007	−0.34	.736	−0.011	−0.59	.556
Personal autonomy				−0.013	−0.70	.482	−0.004	−0.21	.835
Practice location				−0.025	−1.29	.199	−0.026	−1.29	.196
Earnings potential				0.125	4.54	.000	0.123	4.47	.000
Practice setting characteristics									
Kaiser HMO							0.107	1.89	.058
Non-Kaiser group HMO							−0.114	−2.22	.027
Staff HMO							−0.129	−2.25	.024
IPA HMO							−0.014	−0.57	.569
Solo F-F-S							−0.031	−1.52	.130
Intercept	4.087	76.18	.000	4.044	55.88	.000	4.070	44.11	.000
R^2	.238			.245			.249		

Table 4.8 Partial regression and R^2 coefficients, T-ratios, and probability levels obtained from the hierarchical modeling of professional expenses in 1979

	Model 1			Model 2			Model 3		
Variables	b	T-Ratio	Probability Level	b	T-Ratio	Probability Level	b	T-Ratio	Probability Level
Sociodemographic characteristics									
Sex	-0.759	-6.76	.000	-0.738	-6.62	.000	-0.630	-5.96	.000
AMA membership	0.492	9.74	.000	0.495	9.88	.000	0.439	9.20	.000
Board certified	0.209	4.07	.000	0.236	4.61	.000	0.274	5.59	.000
Experience	-0.000	-0.06	.955	-0.000	-0.12	.904	-0.003	-1.44	.150
Internal medicine	-0.041	-0.71	.479	-0.043	-0.75	.454	0.015	0.28	.781
Pediatrics	-0.175	-2.28	.023	-0.167	-2.20	.028	-0.089	-1.22	.222
OB/GYN	.210	2.82	.005	0.197	2.65	.008	0.245	3.49	.001
Environmental characteristics									
Western U.S.	0.061	1.06	.289	0.069	1.21	.225	0.210	3.73	.000
MD/POP ratio	-0.410	-2.52	.012	-0.463	-2.87	.004	-0.355	-2.32	.020
Local income	-0.017	-0.56	.572	-0.014	-0.47	.641	0.007	0.26	.792
Local education	0.013	0.29	.772	0.011	0.24	.807	-0.006	-0.15	.882
Attitudinal characteristics									
Business side				0.208	3.46	.001	0.229	4.03	.000
Scheduling ease				-0.072	-1.35	.178	0.024	0.46	.644
Personal autonomy				0.270	5.54	.000	0.111	2.30	.022
Practice location				-0.108	-2.10	.036	-0.065	-1.33	.183
Earnings potential				0.103	1.45	.146	0.036	0.53	.594
Practice setting characteristics									
Kaiser HMO							-2.388	-12.63	.000
Non-Kaiser group HMO							-1.123	-6.52	.000
Staff HMO							-1.027	-6.57	.000
IPA HMO							0.013	0.22	.828
Solo F-F-S							0.255	5.13	.000
Intercept	3.173	20.10	.000	3.015	17.32	.000	3.069	28.17	.000
R^2	.088			.107			.205		

At the most general level, comparing the R^2 coefficients for models 1, 2, and 3 (see tables 4.7 and 4.8), there is mixed support for the general analytic model. On the one hand, it appears that while the general analytic model does rather well in explaining physician incomes ($R^2 = .249$), the introduction of the practice setting characteristics in model 3 adds only 0.4 percent to the explained variance. Thus, focusing only on the R^2 levels reported in table 4.7 suggests that the practice setting characteristics are virtually unrelated to net physician incomes.

On the other hand, the application of the general analytic model to physicians' professional expenses yields rather robust results. About 20.5 percent of the variance in physician expenses is explained by the sociodemographic, environmental, attitudinal, and practice setting characteristics. Moreover, the introduction of the practice setting characteristics in model 3 increases the explained variance obtained from model 2 by nearly 92 percent. Thus, the data in table 4.8 provide considerable support for our theory, both in terms of the general robustness of the overall model and specifically in terms of the sizable contribution of the practice setting characteristics toward the modeling of physician expenses. Moreover, as we turn to the examination of the effects of each of the sets of the sociodemographic, environmental, attitudinal, and practice setting characteristics on physician incomes, we will find additional support for the effect of the practice setting characteristics.

The effects on physician income of the sociodemographic, environmental, attitudinal, and practice setting characteristics, indicated in the regression coefficients in models 1, 2, and 3 (see table 4.7), are the following. Among the sociodemographic characteristics, all except the dummy variable for pediatrics produced very significant effects on net physician incomes. Moreover, these effects remain virtually unchanged by the introduction of the attitudinal characteristics in model 2 or by the introduction of the practice setting characteristics in model 3. Female physicians have significantly lower net incomes than their male counterparts. This is consistent with the growing literature that has documented the negative effect of being female on physician income (Kehrer 1976; Langwell 1982; Wolinsky and Marder 1983b). Physicians who are members of the AMA have higher net incomes than nonmembers. Similarly, physicians who are board certified have higher incomes than those who are noncertified. The positive effects of AMA membership and board certification probably reflect quality or "seal of approval" designations which justify greater rewards.

At this point, we note that in modeling net physician incomes we have included both the experience variable used in the above analyses and the square of that experience term. The reason is that the effect of experience on income is greatest in the early years of a physician's career, with that effect tapering off as the physician's career peaks. Therefore, we expect a positive experience coefficient, reflecting the greater importance of experience during the earlier career stages, and a negative experience-squared coefficient, reflecting the declining importance of experience during the latter career stages. (See Mincer 1974 and Wolinsky and Marder 1983b for a more detailed discussion of the quadratic modeling techniques used to capture the declining importance of experience on income.) As indicated in table 4.7, the effects of the experience and experience-squared terms are as expected; the experience term produces a significant positive effect, and the experience-squared term produces a significant negative effect.

The effect of the set of dummy variables for medical specialty reveals some interesting observations. Obstetrician/gynecologists have the highest net incomes, followed first by internists and then by general or family practitioners, with pediatricians having lower but not significantly lower incomes than the general or family practitioners. These results are consistent with those typically reported in the literature and reflect the fact that among primary care physicians, obstetrician/gynecologists perform the most surgical procedures and thus have the highest incomes; internists perform more specialized consultations and thus have the next highest incomes.

The environmental characteristics show three interesting points. First, neither the western United States nor local income variables produced statistically significant effects on net physician incomes in any of the three regression models. Thus, physician incomes apparently do not vary across geographic regions, nor are they related to local income levels. The absence of significant effects for these two environmental characteristics is understandable, especially when one considers the fact that third-party insurance payers have probably been responsible for removing geographic and local income fluctuations in physician incomes.

Second is the significant negative effect of the physician-to-population ratio and the local median educational level. The negative physician-to-population ratio effect again indicates that the greater the supply of physicians (and hence the greater the competition), the lower the net income levels. This is intuitively pleasing and provides some evidence for the inelasticity of physician income to physician supply. The significant negative effect of local median educational levels probably means that in more educated areal markets, health status levels are generally higher, and thus the demand for physician services, and consequent physician income, is lower. Third, the regression coefficients obtained for the four variables in model 1 are unaffected by the introduction of the attitudinal characteristics in model 2 and by the addition of the practice setting characteristics in model 3. Thus, the effect of the environmental characteristics is neither spurious to nor suppressed by the attitudinal and practice setting characteristics.

The effects of the attitudinal characteristics on net physician incomes, introduced in model 2, can be described simply. The only attitudinal characteristic that produces a statistically significant effect is the earnings potential variable. Physicians who consider earnings potential to be important in the selection of a practice setting have significantly higher net incomes than do physicians who do not consider it important. This is as expected, and implies that physicians who value

earnings potential manage to obtain higher incomes. As was true for the sociodemographic and environmental characteristics, the effect of earnings potential
is virtually unaltered by the introduction of the practice setting characteristics.

The effects of the practice setting characteristics introduced in model 3 show
additional support for the general analytic model that was not readily observable
by an examination of the R^2 levels alone. As indicated earlier, the introduction
of the practice setting characteristics in model 3 increased the explained variance
by only 0.4 percent. However, as the regression coefficients in table 4.7 indicate,
two of the five practice setting characteristics produced statistically significant
effects on physician incomes, and a third characteristic's effect almost reached
statistical significance. Physicians in non-Kaiser group model HMOs and in staff
model HMOs have significantly lower net incomes than their group fee-for-service
counterparts. This supports the growing literature (see Fink 1980) suggesting that
one of the reasons for the difficulties in recruiting physicians into HMOs is the
significantly lower salaries that they will receive there. However, while the effect
of the Kaiser model HMO variable is not quite statistically significant, it indicates
that physicians in this practice setting have higher net incomes than those in group
fee-for-service.

These findings raise two important issues. First, they suggest that rather
than receiving lower incomes than their group fee-for-service counterparts, physicians in Kaiser model HMOs may actually receive higher incomes. Second, the
negative and statistically significant effect of the non-Kaiser group model HMO
variable, coupled with the positive but not quite statistically significant effect for
the Kaiser model HMO variable, indicates further the considerable importance
of distinguishing between traditional Kaiser model HMOs and the hybrid PPD/FFS
model HMOs suggested by Krill and Gaynor (1982) and Wolinsky and Marder
(1982a). Indeed, the separation of the Kaiser model HMO physicians from the
non-Kaiser group model HMO physicians may explain why in our early analyses
of these same data we failed to find a statistically significant effect (either positive
or negative) for the more grossly measured group model (i.e., both Kaiser and
non-Kaiser) HMO variable (see Wolinsky and Marder 1983b).

Another intriguing finding is the absence of a statistically significant effect
for the solo fee-for-service variable. Researchers have traditionally found that physicians in solo fee-for-service practice have significantly lower incomes than their
group fee-for-service counterparts. In our more precise modeling of physician net
incomes herein, where we include a number of measures of the sociodemographic,
environmental, and attitudinal characteristics in addition to the practice setting
characteristics, we do not find the net incomes of solo fee-for-service physicians
to be significantly different from those in group fee-for-service practice. This suggests either that further research on the income of solo versus group practice fee-
for-service physicians is in order or that the traditional differentials between them
no longer exist.

The results obtained from models 1, 2, and 3 in predicting physicians' professional expenses are shown in table 4.8. Among the sociodemographic characteristics the results indicate that female physicians report having significantly fewer professional expenses than their male counterparts. While the introduction of the attitudinal characteristics in model 2 does not diminish this effect, the introduction of the practice setting characteristics in model 3 does. However, even after the introduction of the practice setting characteristics, female physicians continue to report lower professional expenses.

Members of the AMA report significantly greater professional expenses than non-AMA members; the same is true for board certified physicians versus non-board certified physicians. The greater professional expenses associated with being a member of the AMA and being board certified in part reflect the membership fees of these professional societies. However, the increased professional expenses far exceed those membership fees and probably include other investments in human capital such as continuing education, professional journals, and attendance at professional meetings. All of these activities are likely to be more common for members of the AMA and for board certified physicians.

The experience term fails to produce a statistically significant effect on professional expenses in any of the three regression models. Accordingly, it appears that professional expenses are relatively constant across a physician's career. This seems reasonable.

The effect of the set of dummy variables for medical specialty on professional expenses produces interesting results. Only the regression coefficient for obstetrics/gynecology is statistically significant in the presence of the practice setting characteristics. The effect of pediatrics is statistically significant until the practice setting characteristics are introduced; it is then reduced to insignificance. The dummy variable for internal medicine never produces a statistically significant effect in any of the three regression models. When taken together, these data indicate that internists, pediatricians, and general or family practitioners do not have significantly more or less professional expense than each other. However, obstetrician/gynecologists have significantly more professional expenses than these physicians. Their greater professional expenses probably reflect the additional costs of providing surgical services to their patients.

Three interesting facts emerge from the effects of the environmental characteristics on professional expenses. First, neither local income nor median educational levels ever produces statistically significant effects on professional expenses. This indicates that professional expenses are unrelated to patient characteristics. While this may seem counter-intuitive, we remind the reader that "bad debts" in particular are not included within the realm of professional expenses. This may, in part, explain why professional expenses appear unrelated to patient characteristics.

Second, although the western United States variable does not have a significant effect on professional expenses in either model 1 or model 2, the introduction of the practice setting characteristics in model 3 changes the situation. In the presence of the practice setting characteristics, the western United States variable has a significant positive effect on professional expenses. That is, physicians in the western United States report having higher levels of professional expenses than their nonwestern counterparts, although this relationship does not emerge until the practice setting characteristics are brought into the equation.

The third interesting finding among the environmental characteristics is that the physician-to-population ratio produces a statistically significant negative effect on professional expenses in all three of the regression models. Moreover, although the magnitude of the effect fluctuates somewhat, it is not significantly altered by the introduction of either the attitudinal or practice setting characteristics. The negative effect of the physician-to-population ratio indicates that the greater the supply of physicians relative to the population (i.e., the greater the competition), the lower the physician's professional expenses. This suggests that increased competition somehow reduces professional expenses, perhaps as a result of streamlining operations in the presence of price competition. Further research on this issue, however, is needed before this interpretation can be considered more than speculative.

When the attitudinal characteristics are introduced in model 2, three of them produce statistically significant effects on professional expenses. Both the business side of practice and personal autonomy variables have significant positive effects on professional expenses, while the practice location variable has a significant negative effect. Thus, physicians for whom the business side of practice was an important issue in selecting a practice setting report greater professional expenses than those who found it less important. Physicians who value personal autonomy in selecting a practice setting also report higher professional expenses. Finally, physicians who consider the practice location issue very important in selecting a practice setting report having lower professional expenses.

The practice setting characteristics introduced in model 3 yield considerable support for our general theoretical perspective. The dummy variables representing all three of the closed-panel type of HMOs (Kaiser model, non-Kaiser group model, and staff model) have statistically significant negative effects on professional expenses. Thus, physicians in Kaiser model HMOs, non-Kaiser group model HMOs, and staff model HMOs have significantly lower professional expenses than their group fee-for-service counterparts. Moreover, among the physicians in these closed-panel model HMOs, Kaiser model HMO physicians have the lowest professional expenses, followed by physicians in non-Kaiser group model HMOs, with physicians in staff model HMOs having the highest level of professional expenses of physicians in closed-panel model HMOs. Physicians in IPA model HMOs have professional expenses that are neither significantly greater nor less than in group fee-for-service, precisely as our theory suggests.

Finally, the data in table 4.8 indicate that physicians in solo fee-for-service practices have significantly greater levels of professional expenses than their group fee-for-service counterparts. Indeed, those in solo fee-for-service practice have the highest level of professional expenses of physicians in any of the six practice settings. This is also as expected, especially given that in any group practice arrangement professional expenses are more likely to be absorbed by the corporation than by the individual physician.

Although tables 4.7 and 4.8 present the precise effects on physician incomes and professional expenses for each of the variables in our general analytic model, they do not intuitively portray the magnitude of the differences in physician incomes and professional expenses across the various organizational forms of medical practice. To compensate for these shortcomings, we have again used the precise effects of the general analytic model to adjust physician incomes and professional expenses within each of the six practice settings for differences in the sociodemographic, environmental, and attitudinal characteristics. Table 4.9 shows the results of these calculations. The data in table 4.9 flesh out a more intuitively pleasing demonstration of the support for our theory than can be obtained solely from the hierarchical regression results of the natural logarithms of physician incomes and professional expenses presented in tables 4.7 and 4.8.

Summary and Discussion

A considerable amount of information has been presented from the complex statistical analyses that were reported in this chapter. The most effective way to summarize and discuss these results is to focus on the four important points that have emerged concerning how the organization of medical practice affects the practice of medicine. The first relates to the hierarchical modeling of the total

Table 4.9   Average adjusted means for physician income and expenses by practice setting

Practice Setting	Physician Income	Professional Expenses
Kaiser model HMO	72.3	3.0
Non-Kaiser group model HMO	58.0	10.6
Staff model HMO	57.1	11.6
IPA model HMO	64.1	32.0
Group F-F-S	65.0	32.4
Solo F-F-S	63.0	41.8

Note: Means are expressed in thousands of dollars and are adjusted for differences in the sociodemographic, environmental, and attitudinal characteristics used in the general analytic model.

number of hours worked per week and the number of direct patient care hours worked per week. The regression coefficients shown in tables 4.2 and 4.3 clearly indicate that the organization of medical practice does not affect either of these two measures of the general volume of physicians' weekly workloads. That is, there are no differences in the general weekly workload between physicians practicing in any of the six practice settings. This is not necessarily devastating for our theory; rather, what it indicates most is that physicians from all practice settings practice medicine about the same number of hours per week, both overall and in direct patient care. Thus, these data suggest that, at least with respect to practice setting characteristics, the overall volume of physicians' weekly workloads is apparently standard.

The second point emerges from the hierarchical modeling of how physicians distribute that apparently standard weekly workload between seeing patients in the office and in the hospital. The analysis of the internal distribution of office and hospital visits provides considerable support for (1) our theoretical orientation that this distribution is very closely related to practice setting characteristics, and (2) the extant explanation that this is how HMOs attain their cost savings. These two issues are extraordinarily intertwined. The regression coefficients shown in tables 4.4 and 4.5 indicate that physicians in Kaiser model HMOs, the archetypical closed-panel HMO, had an average of slightly more than 22 more office visits per week than their counterparts in group fee-for-service. At the same time, physicians in Kaiser model HMOs had an average of about 8 fewer hospital visits than did those in group fee-for-service. Similar differentials were observed by comparing non-Kaiser group model HMO physicians with group fee-for-service physicians. Thus, these data provide considerable support for the argument that HMOs, especially group model HMOs, achieve their cost savings by providing more ambulatory care coupled with less hospital-based care (see Luft 1978a, 1978b, 1981, 1983; Wolinsky 1980).

These data also provide considerable support for the previous arguments of Wolinsky and his colleagues (see Wolinsky 1980; Wolinsky and Corry 1981; Wolinsky and Marder 1982a, 1982b, 1983a, 1983b) that physicians in IPA model HMOs do not practice medicine differently from their counterparts in group fee-for-service practice. That is, the dummy variable for IPA model HMOs failed to produce statistically significant effects on either the number of office visits or the number of hospital visits. Overall, then, the analysis of the office and hospital visit data clearly demonstrates that this significant aspect of physician workload characteristics is very much related to the organization of medical practice.

Third, considerable support was provided for our theory by the modeling of physician net incomes, as several of the practice setting characteristics produced statistically significant effects on net physician incomes. There were two very interesting and different trends in these results. On the one hand, the regression coefficients shown in table 4.7 demonstrate that non-Kaiser group model HMO and staff model HMO physicians have significantly lower net incomes than their group fee-for-service counterparts, or for that matter, than their counterparts in IPA model HMOs or in solo fee-for-service practices. This is consistent with prior speculation (cf. Fink 1980), which has traditionally suggested that physicians in HMOs receive lower incomes and that this accounts for the difficulty of recruiting physicians into HMOs.

On the other hand, although not statistically significant at the .05 level (but at the .058 level), the regression coefficient for physicians in Kaiser model HMOs indicates that their net incomes are considerably higher than those in group fee-for-service practices. Moreover, these data indicate that the net incomes of physicians in Kaiser model HMOs are higher than those of physicians in all of the five other practice settings. This finding is not consistent with the existing literature and thus should be replicated before it is fully and openly accepted. Nonetheless, this finding does demonstrate the crucial importance of distinguishing between traditional Kaiser model HMOs and the new hybrid non-Kaiser group model HMOs. As Krill and Gaynor (1982) suggest, these data indicate that there are very real differences between the traditional and hybrid group model HMOs.

Fourth, concerning the effect of the organization of medical practice on professional expenses, the results of the regression coefficients for the practice setting characteristics shown in table 4.8 are quite consistent with our expectations. The professional expenses of physicians in the three closed-panel HMOs (i.e., Kaiser model, non-Kaiser group model, and staff model) are significantly lower than those of group fee-for-service physicians. In addition, once again we find that physicians in IPA model (i.e., open-panel) HMOs have professional expense levels no different from those of their group fee-for-service counterparts. Finally, the data indicate that physicians in solo fee-for-service practice have the highest level of professional expenses of physicians in any of the six practice settings. These results are as we had expected. The more bureaucratic the practice setting, the more likely it is that the corporation, as opposed to the individual physician, will absorb professional expenses. Thus, solo fee-for-service practitioners have the highest professional expense levels, and physicians in Kaiser model HMOs have the lowest. Indeed, there is a perfect fit between our theoretical expectations expressed in figure 1.5 and the ordering of professional expenses shown in table 4.8. Thus, the analysis of the professional expense data also provide considerable support for our theory.

References

Fink, Ray. 1980. "HMO physicians' recruitment stymied by higher fee-for-service salaries." *Group Health News* 21:8–9.

Freidson, Eliot. 1970. *Profession of Medicine: A Study of the Sociology of Applied Knowledge.*

New York: Harper and Row.

Kehrer, Barbara. 1976. "Factors affecting the incomes of men and women physicians: An exploratory study." *Journal of Human Resources* 11:526–39.

Krill, Mary, and Ralph Gaynor. 1982. "An assessment of the future of HMOs." *Medical Group Management* 29:42–46.

Langwell, Kathryn. 1982. "Factors affecting the incomes of men and women physicians: Further explorations." *Journal of Human Resources* 17:261–74.

Luft, Harold. 1978a. "How do health maintenance organizations achieve their savings? Rhetoric and evidence." *New England Journal of Medicine* 298:1336–43.

_____. 1978b. "Why do HMOs seem to provide more health maintenance services?" *Milbank Memorial Fund Quarterly* 56:140–68.

_____. 1981. *Health Maintenance Organizations: Dimensions of Performance.* New York: Wiley.

_____. 1983. "Health maintenance organizations." In *Handbook of Health, Health Care, and the Health Professions,* edited by David Mechanic. New York: Free Press.

Mincer, Jacob. 1974. *Schooling, Experience, and Earnings.* New York: National Bureau of Economic Research.

Wolinsky, Fredric. 1980. "The performance of health maintenance organizations: An analytic review." *Milbank Memorial Fund Quarterly* 58:537–82.

Wolinsky, Fredric, and Barbara Corry. 1981. "Organizational structure and medical practice in health maintenance organizations." In *Profile of Medical Practice, 1981,* edited by David Goldfarb. Chicago: American Medical Association.

Wolinsky, Fredric, and William Marder. 1982a. "HMOs: The concept, new evidence and implications." *Medical Group Management* 29:50–52, 58.

_____. 1982b. "Spending time with patients: The impact of organizational structure on medical practice." *Medical Care* 20:1051–59.

_____. 1983a. "Waiting to see the doctor: The impact of organizational structure on medical practice." *Medical Care* 21:531–42.

_____. 1983b. "The organization of medical practice and primary care physician income." *American Journal of Public Health* 73:379–82.

5

Toward a Theory of the Organization of Medical Practice and the Practice of Medicine

Overview

The purpose of this chapter is fourfold. First, we review the relationships that we expected between the organization of medical practice and the practice of medicine. Second, we summarize the actual relationships that were observed and present three possible caveats concerning the interpretation of those relationships. Third, we present the modifications of our theory that are necessary and appropriate in light of the relationships observed in our sample of 3,555 primary care physicians. In particular, these modifications focus on greater specificity for the effects of the organization of medical practice on the different dimensions of the practice of medicine. Finally, we discuss the major policy implications that both our theory and our findings have for the American health care delivery system. In particular, we consider how our work might influence national policies designed to maximize the quality of health care and minimize its cost.

What We Expected

To review the general outline of our theory of the relationship between the organization of medical practice and the practice of medicine, refer to figure 1.5. As the reader will recall, figure 1.5 portrayed the ordering and approximate relative placement of the six practice settings on the autonomous-bureaucratic dimension of medical practice that underlies most discussions of the organization of medical practice. Figure 1.5, reproduced here as figure 5.1, shows that the six practice settings we have examined can be placed along the medical practice continuum between the autonomous end and the bureaucratic end. According to our theory,

Figure 5.1   Ordering and approximate relative placement of the six practice settings on the autonomous-bureaucratic continuum of medical practice

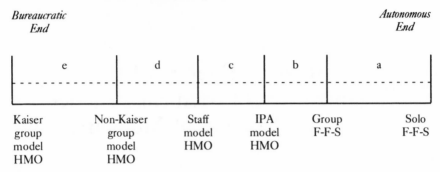

| *Bureaucratic End* | | | | | *Autonomous End* |

| e | d | c | b | a |

| Kaiser group model HMO | Non-Kaiser group model HMO | Staff model HMO | IPA model HMO | Group F-F-S | Solo F-F-S |

from autonomous to bureaucratic (i.e., from right to left) one encounters, in order, solo fee-for-service practices, group fee-for-service practices, IPA model HMOs, staff model HMOs, non-Kaiser group model HMOs, and Kaiser model HMOs. The distances between any two contiguous practice settings in figure 5.1 are indicated by the space occupied by the letters *a* through *e*.

At the most general level, we expected there would be changes in the practice of medicine (with the one exception of the special case of the IPA model HMO) as one moved from the more autonomous end of the continuum to the more bureaucratic end. For example, it has long been assumed and documented that the practice of medicine in solo fee-for-service settings is different from that in group fee-for-service settings. Thus, we expected the difference between these two practice settings, denoted by the letter *a*, to be significant. We did not expect, however, to find any significant differences between the practice of medicine in group fee-for-service practices and IPA model HMOs; thus, we expected the distance represented by the letter *b* to be insignificant. We expected the practice of medicine in group fee-for-service settings and in IPA model HMOs to be similar because physicians in both practice settings face the same organizational and fiscal incentive structures. Thus, we would not normally expect them to practice medicine differently from each other.

The differences between all of the other practice settings, as represented by the letters *c* through *e*, were thought to be significant. Therefore, we expected that the practice of medicine in staff model HMOs would be different from that in any of the five other practice settings. Similarly, we expected that the practice of medicine in non-Kaiser group model HMOs would be different from that in any of the other five practice settings. Finally, we expected that the practice of medicine in Kaiser model HMOs would be different from that in any of the other five practice settings.

We also expected that there would be a relatively consistent pattern of differences between the six practice settings. For example, in examining the effects of the organization of medical practice on the amount of time spent with patients, we expected that longer patient visits would be associated with the practice settings at the more autonomous end of the continuum, and shorter patient visits with the practice settings at the more bureaucratic end of the continuum. This expectation was derived from Freidson's (1970) classic work on the client dependency of physicians in solo practice versus the colleague dependency of physicians in more bureaucratic settings. These expectations are also consistent with Mechanic's (1975) "target-time" hypothesis suggesting that, when faced with increased patient demands for physician services, physicians in solo fee-for-service practice settings would respond by working longer hours so that they could accommodate all of their patients with the traditional visit length. Mechanic hypothesized that physicians in prepaid group practices would respond to increased demands for patient services by spending less time per patient, so that they would have to work only the same number of hours.

As a corollary to our expectations concerning the amount of time spent per patient, we anticipated that patient queues would show the reverse ordering. We expected that patients who saw solo fee-for-service physicians would have the shortest queues, while their counterparts who received care from physicians in the most bureaucratic practice settings would have the longest queues. This expectation is also consistent with Freidson's (1970), Mechanic's (1975), and Held and Reinhardt's (1979) work suggesting that especially in prepaid practice settings, patient queues are used as a nonprice rationing device to maintain patients' demands for physician services at a manageable level.

For both sets of expectations (time spent with patients and patient queues), we predicted that the relative ordering of the six practice settings shown in figure 5.1 would be observed. The amount of time spent per patient would be highest in the solo fee-for-service practice setting and would monotonically decline until it reached its lowest point in Kaiser model HMOs. Conversely, we predicted that the lag time for appointments to see a physician would be greatest in Kaiser model HMOs and would then monotonically decline until it reached its lowest level in solo fee-for-service practice settings.

Our expectations concerning the relationships between physician workload characteristics and the organization of medical practice were somewhat different and not nearly so well specified. On the one hand, we did not expect gross physician workload characteristics, such as the total number of hours worked per week or the number of direct patient care hours, to be related to the organization of medical practice. Indeed, no previous literature had suggested that the total number of hours worked per week would vary by practice setting. Thus, there was insufficient prior evidence and conjecture upon which to base specific expectations for a pattern of relationships between the organization of medical practice and gross physician workload characteristics. On the other hand, sufficient evidence and conjecture led us to predict relationships between the organization of medical practice and the number of office visits and hospital visits encountered per week.

In particular, the literature assessing the performance of HMOs strongly suggests that HMOs may achieve their cost savings by substituting ambulatory care for hospital-based services (see Luft 1978a, 1978b, 1980, 1981, 1983). Therefore, although we did not expect to see variations in the total number of hours worked per week, we did expect to see more ambulatory care visits coupled with fewer hospital-based visits in HMO practice settings than in non-HMO practice settings. Moreover, given that the incentive structure which would support substitution effects is maximized in Kaiser model HMOs and minimized in staff model HMOs (with non-Kaiser group model HMOs falling somewhere in between), we expected the substitution effects to increase in magnitude, along the autonomous-bureaucratic continuum, from staff model HMOs to non-Kaiser group model HMOs and finally to Kaiser model HMOs.

Finally, turning to the issues of physician incomes and professional expenses, we expected the following. Although there was not a well-developed empirical literature concerning physician incomes in HMOs, some polemical writings suggest that physicians in HMOs make less money than their counterparts in group fee-for-service practice settings. Indeed, the alleged income gap between HMO physicians and their better paid non-HMO counterparts has been touted as one of the major obstacles in the recruitment of physicians into HMOs (Fink 1980). Accordingly, there was sufficient speculation to lead us to expect that physicians in HMOs would receive lower incomes than their non-HMO counterparts. However, the available data was not sufficient to warrant further speculation on how the salaries of physicians in the different types of HMOs would compare with each other.

Our expectations concerning physicians' professional expenses are both more and less straightforward than those concerning physicians' incomes. On the one hand, because literature on physicians' professional expenses is virtually nonexistent (cf. Held and Reinhardt 1979), we have little on which to base our expectations. On the other hand, it seems intuitively pleasing that, as one moves from the autonomous end to the bureaucratic end of the continuum, it is more likely that the corporate entity will absorb the professional expenses of the physicians in its employ. Thus, it seems plausible to expect that physicians' professional expenses would be at their greatest levels in solo fee-for-service settings and would decline in a monotonic fashion toward the bureaucratic end of the continuum, with the least professional expenses in Kaiser model HMOs. That is, it would seem that the more bureaucratic the medical practice, the more likely that the organization would absorb physicians' professional expenses.

What We Found

Having reviewed what we expected, we now turn to a review of what we found concerning the effects of the organization of medical practice on the practice of medicine. The effects of the practice setting characteristics on the amount of time it takes for new and established patients to schedule a routine office visit were perfectly consistent with our expectations. Patient queues were arrayed from longest to shortest in this order: Kaiser model HMOs, non-Kaiser group model HMOs, staff model HMOs, IPA model HMOs, group fee-for-service practices, and solo fee-for-service practices. Moreover, we expected that all six practice settings would have patient queues significantly different from each other, with the exception of the patient queues in IPA model HMOs (we anticipated them to be the same as those in group fee-for-service practices). The results obtained from the hierarchical modeling of appointment scheduling times fit this hierarchical sequence precisely, with the IPA model physicians imposing the same patient queues as their group fee-for-service counterparts. Thus, what we found was exactly what we had expected: the more bureaucratic the practice setting, the longer the patient scheduling queues.

Although the effects of the practice setting characteristics on patient scheduling queues supported our theory, this was not true for the effects on waiting room queues. The results of the hierarchical modeling of waiting room queues showed that Kaiser model HMOs, non-Kaiser group model HMOs, and solo fee-for-service practice settings had significantly shorter waiting room queues than their group fee-for-service counterparts. While we had expected patients of physicians in solo fee-for-service practice settings to have shorter waiting room queues than those who saw physicians in group fee-for-service practices (due to the greater client dependency in solo fee-for-service practice), we had expected patients in all of the closed-panel model HMOs to face longer patient waiting room queues; that was not the case. Moreover, the results showed that waiting room queues in solo fee-for-service practice, Kaiser model HMOs, and non-Kaiser group model HMOs were about the same. This, of course, contradicts not only our theory but also previous literature containing hypotheses that physicians in prepaid group practices would use both scheduling and waiting room queues as nonprice rationing devices to maintain patient demand levels at a manageable level (see Held and Reinhardt 1979).

The effect of the practice setting characteristics on the amount of time spent per patient in the office yields considerable support for our theory, as the results of the hierarchical modeling are almost exactly as we had expected. Physicians in solo fee-for-service practice have the longest patient visits, followed in order by physicians in group fee-for-service practice, IPA model HMOs, staff model HMOs, non-Kaiser group model HMOs, and Kaiser model HMOs. In addition, the results also indicate that office visit lengths among IPA model HMO physicians are not significantly different from those of their group fee-for-service practice counterparts. The only element that did not completely support our expectations was the effect of being in a staff model HMO. Although the length of office visits with staff model HMO physicians fit into the expected monotonic decline from the autonomous end to the bureaucratic end of medical practice, the length of their office visits was not significantly different from that of their group fee-for-service counterparts. Nonetheless, the hierarchical modeling of office visit lengths did provide considerable support for our theory.

Less support was provided by the hierarchical modeling of hospital visit lengths. We had expected the same monotonic relationship between the six practice settings and hospital visit lengths that we had expected and observed for office visit lengths. However, only for physicians in staff model HMOs and in solo fee-for-service practices were hospital visit lengths significantly different from those in group fee-for-service practice. These results indicated that solo fee-for-service physicians spent more time per patient in the hospital than group fee-for-service physicians, and that staff model HMO physicians spent the most time. Thus, the results of the hierarchical modeling of hospital visit lengths did not provide much support for our theory.

Using the general analytic model to hierarchically predict the gross measures of physician workload characteristics also failed to support our theory. None of the practice setting characteristics produced statistically significant effects on either the total number of hours that physicians worked per week or the number of hours in direct patient care that they provided per week. Thus, there appears to be a "normal" work week, the length of which is unrelated to the organization of medical practice.

The two measures of how the practice of medicine is distributed within that "normal" work week, however, did support our theory. When we used the hierarchical modeling process to predict separately the number of office visits and the number of hospital visits, we observed the expected effects of the organization of medical practice. Physicians in Kaiser model HMOs had significantly more office visits and significantly fewer hospital visits per week than their counterparts in group fee-for-service practice. Similarly (although this is not quite statistically significant), physicians in non-Kaiser group model HMOs had more office visits than those in group fee-for-service; they had significantly fewer hospital visits per week than those in group fee-for-service. Thus, these data supported our expectation that, at least in the archetypical prepaid group practices (Kaiser and non-Kaiser group model HMOs), there is considerable evidence that ambulatory care is substituted for hospital-based services.

The relationship between the organization of medical practice and physician incomes also provided somewhat mixed support for our theory. Non-Kaiser group model HMOs and staff model HMOs yielded significantly lower net incomes than group fee-for-service. That result was consistent with our expectations based upon the growing literature suggesting that one of the reasons for the difficulty in recruiting physicians into HMOs is the significantly lower salaries they will receive. Although not quite statistically significantly different, physicians in Kaiser model HMOs had higher net incomes than their group fee-for-service counterparts. Another unexpected finding was the similarity between the incomes of physicians in solo and group fee-for-service practices. Traditionally it has been assumed that solo fee-for-service physicians earn less than those in group fee-for-service practice. Our results indicate that the difference is not enough to be statistically significant. Overall, then, the analyses of physicians' incomes provided somewhat mixed support for our theory on the effects of the organization of medical practice; although there are significant differences in net incomes between several of the practice settings, those differences were not entirely as we had expected.

Finally, the hierarchical modeling of physicians' professional expenses provided considerable support for our general theoretical perspective. All three of the closed-panel HMO types had significantly lower professional expenses than group fee-for-service practice. Moreover, among the physicians in the closed-panel model HMOs, Kaiser model HMO physicians had the lowest professional expenses, followed by physicians in non-Kaiser group model HMOs, while physicians in staff model HMOs had the highest expenses. Also consistently with our theory, physicians in IPA model HMOs had professional expenses neither significantly greater nor less than their group fee-for-service counterparts. Again, as we had expected, physicians in solo fee-for-service practice had the highest level of professional expenses of physicians in any of the six practice settings. Thus, the relationship between the organization of medical practice and physicians' professional expenses was exactly as we had expected.

Before we consider modifying our theory in light of these relationships, there are three caveats concerning the data that should be reviewed. The first concerns the general reliability and validity of the data on physicians obtained from PSP–14. This was discussed at some length in chapter 2, and we shall not repeat our defense of these data here in its entirety. The basic issues here are whether these data are reliable and valid for assessing the effects of the organization of medical practice on the practice of medicine. Given the manner in which the PSP data in general, and the PSP–14 data in particular, are gathered, it is not possible to assess directly the reliability of the measures used here. However, a variety of other indirect methods for assessing the reliability of the PSP–14 data have been used, as reported in chapter 2. Based on these indirect assessments, we believe that the PSP–14 data are sufficiently reliable both to warrant our analyses and support our conclusions.

The validity of the data from PSP–14 was also discussed in chapter 2. Recall that our argument for the validity of using these data to assess the effect of the organization of medical practice on the practice of medicine focuses not on the point estimates themselves (i.e., average patient queues, time spent with patients, incomes, and so forth), but on the differences between the point estimates obtained for physicians across the six practice settings. As indicated in chapter 2, there is no evidence to suggest that an analysis of the differences in those point estimates would be invalid. Accordingly, although the reliability and validity issues surrounding the PSP–14 data have not and cannot be definitively resolved, we believe that these data are appropriate for the purposes of this research.

The second caveat concerns the five measures of attitudinal characteristics. We would have preferred to have a more elaborate set of measures of physicians' attitudes on the self-selection issues. We would rather have taken these measurements at the time when physicians actually chose their practice settings. That, however, was not possible. Accordingly, these measures of the attitudinal characteristics probably contain some amount of measurement error. Nonetheless, because we are using these proxy measures of physicians' attitudes to adjust for potential self-selection effects, and because we do not focus on these effects as the principal tests of our hypotheses, we do not believe that the potential measurement error jeopardizes our conclusions. Indeed, as potentially gross as they may be, our inclusion of these proxy measures of physicians' attitudes represents the first attempt by research in this area to adjust for the self-selection issue.

Third is the absence of data on the sociodemographic, environmental, and attitudinal characteristics of the patients who went to the physicians in our sample. This issue was discussed in chapter 1. We indicated that although none of these characteristics was directly measured at the patient's level, there would be a close correspondence between the practice setting characteristics for the physician and the patient, as well as between the environmental characteristics for the physician and the patient. However, the sociodemographic and attitudinal characteristics of the patient and the physician would not be expected to overlap as closely, although one could assume that patients and physicians with similar attitudes would be attracted to each other.

There is no technique that can be used with any certainty to dispel the possibility that the absence of the direct measurement of patient characteristics may have contaminated our results. At the same time, however, there is no evidence suggesting that this absence jeopardizes our findings. Rather, it seems most likely that it would simply attenuate the observed relationships between the organization of medical practice and the practice of medicine. Therefore, in a more completely specified (i.e., doubly-subscripted) version of the general analytic model, we might anticipate finding stronger relationships between the organization of medical practice and the practice of medicine.

Modifying the Theory in Light of the Findings

Given the relationships between the organization of medical practice and the practice of medicine that were and were not observed in the analyses of our sample of 3,555 primary care physicians, some modifications in our basic theory are warranted at this point. In particular, there are five areas in which such modifications are both straightforward and appropriate: (1) waiting room queues, (2) hospital visit lengths, (3) gross workload characteristics, (4) substitution of ambulatory for hospital-based services, and (5) net incomes.

Contrary to our expectations, waiting room queues were not the shortest in solo fee-for-service practice, and they did not increase in a monotonic fashion across the more bureaucratic forms of medical practice. Indeed, waiting room queues significantly differed from those found in group fee-for-service practices only for Kaiser model HMOs, non-Kaiser group model HMOs, and solo fee-for-service practice settings. Moreover, the magnitude of the regression coefficients for these dummy variables suggested that in these three practice settings patients waited about the same amount of time in the office. Thus, our data actually show that the shortest waiting room queues occurred at both ends of the autonomous-bureaucratic continuum. This is clearly not consistent with our expectations or with those of other economically-based theories that expect closed-panel HMOs to manipulate waiting room queues as a nonprice rationing device in order to arrive at and maintain manageable levels of patient demands (see especially Held and Reinhardt 1979; Mechanic 1975). This anomalous finding represents perhaps the most contradictory evidence for our general theoretical perspective.

There is a potentially viable, albeit ad hoc, explanation for these apparently aberrant findings. The waiting room queue results may actually indicate an explicit attempt by physicians and practice managers in Kaiser and non-Kaiser group model HMOs to offset the "clinic" atmosphere that has generally been attributed to their practice settings (see Berki and Ashcraft 1980). The literature reviewed in chapter 1 indicates that the American public traditionally has viewed prepaid group practices as relatively synonymous with "public clinics." Public clinics, of course, are not the site of choice. One of the most common complaints about public clinics is the incredibly long delay in seeing a physician. Such delays are typically spent in overcrowded and not very desirable waiting rooms. Allegedly, many people associate both the longer waiting room queues and the more unpleasant waiting room environment of public clinics with those in closed-panel HMO settings. Accordingly, physicians and practice managers in Kaiser and non-Kaiser group model HMOs may concentrate on reducing waiting room queues in order to improve their public image and create the impression of providing medical care (as expressed by waiting room queues) that is indistinguishable from that found in solo fee-for-service practice.

Although this interpretation appears to be straightforward and reasonable, it clearly implies a concerted effort by physicians and practice managers in Kaiser and non-Kaiser group model HMOs. Unfortunately, there is no way for us to document the existence of this concerted effort by means of the PSP–14 data. Support for this interpretation, however, can be gleaned by examining the waiting room queues of patients seeing physicians in staff model and IPA model HMOs:

their waiting room queues are not significantly different from those found in group fee-for-service practice settings. The similarity of IPA model HMO waiting room queues to those in group fee-for-service practice settings was explicitly anticipated in our theory. Although unanticipated, it is nevertheless intuitively pleasing that waiting room queues in staff model HMOs are similar to those found in group fee-for-service practice, especially when one considers that physicians in staff model HMOs do not have a proprietary interest in the HMO. Thus, they are less likely to actively participate in the reduction of waiting room queues in order to enhance the image of the HMO.

When taken together, the results of the hierarchical modeling of waiting room queues prompts us to suggest the following modification of our theory. We now expect future studies of the relationship between the organization of medical practice and waiting room queues to identify shorter queues for patients in solo fee-for-service practices, Kaiser model HMOs, and non-Kaiser group model HMOs. At the same time, we expect future studies to find that waiting room queues in the three other practice settings would be approximately equal to each other and longer than those in either solo fee-for-service practice, Kaiser model HMOs, or non-Kaiser group model HMOs.

The second area where modification of our theory seems appropriate involves the relationship between the organization of medical practice and hospital visit lengths. Only the staff model HMO and the solo fee-for-service practice setting variables produced statistically significant effects. As expected, solo fee-for-service physicians spent more time per patient in the hospital than their group fee-for-service counterparts. Physicians in staff model HMOs, however, spent even more time per patient in the hospital than solo fee-for-service physicians. This latter result is quite inconsistent with our theory. Also unexpected is the absence of effects of being in either Kaiser model or non-Kaiser group model HMOs. In short, the analysis of hospital visit lengths did not produce results consistent with our expectations.

At this point we are prepared to modify this part of our theory. Rather than attempting to recast our theory to compensate for these anomalous findings, we now submit that our original theory overstated the potential impact of the organization of medical practice on hospital visit lengths. It was, perhaps, overzealous of us to assume that the effects of the six practice settings specified herein, which are basically *office* practice settings, would carry over into the practice of medicine in the hospital setting. Although the data did demonstrate a consistent relationship between the organization of medical practice and office visit lengths, this relationship did not spill over into hospital visit lengths, nor was there much reason for us to have expected that it would.

Basically, our theory argued that the practice of medicine in IPA model HMOs would not significantly differ from that in group fee-for-service practice settings. The reason was that the "prepaid incentives" operative in IPA model

HMOs constituted a very small portion of IPA model physicians' practices, and thus were not likely to affect their nonprepaid practices. Similarly, it may have been a logical error for us to expect spillover effects for the organization of medical practice into the practice of medicine in the hospital setting for two reasons. First, the ratio of office visits to hospital visits among the primary care physicians in our sample was about 4:1, indicating that the vast majority of medical practice occurs in the office setting. Thus, hospital practice may be relatively unaffected by the organization of the office practice setting. Second, only Kaiser model HMO physicians face the full-time effects of prepaid medicine in an integrated organizational system. Thus, if physicians in any form of an HMO were to have shorter hospital visit lengths, they should be Kaiser model HMO physicians. Although not quite statistically significant, this was the case; Kaiser model HMO physicians had hospital visit lengths about 4.2 minutes shorter, on average, than their counterparts in group fee-for-service practice settings.

Based on the above, we expect that future studies of the relationship between the organization of medical practice and hospital visit lengths will find only one or two significant effects. First, physicians in solo fee-for-service practices will have the longest hospital visit lengths, due to the increased patient dependency of physicians in this practice setting. Second, if any practice setting has hospital visit lengths shorter than those in group fee-for-service practice, we expect it to be Kaiser model HMOs. There, medicine is practiced full time in a prepaid environment designed to maximize physicians' cost-containment incentives.

The third area in which a modification of our theoretical perspective appears both straightforward and appropriate involves the relationship between the organization of medical practice and gross workload characteristics. As indicated in the analyses presented in chapter 4, there were no significant relationships between the organization of medical practice and gross workload characteristics among physicians in any of the six practice settings. Indeed, the results presented herein appear to suggest that a standard work week exists, at least among primary care physicians. Moreover, this standard work week is not significantly affected by our measures of the six practice settings, although both the total number of hours worked per week and the number of hours spent in direct patient care tended to be slightly less in the three closed-panel types of HMOs.

This actually seems intuitively pleasing, indicating that it is not by working more hours in general that physicians achieve or fail to achieve cost effectiveness, but that such achievements lie in how the standard work week is spent. Accordingly, we expect that future studies of the relationship between the organization of medical practice and physician workload characteristics will not find significant differences in the total number of hours worked per week or the number of hours of direct patient care provided. Rather, we assume that future studies will replicate our identification of a standard work week for primary care physicians, regardless of the particular setting in which they practice medicine.

The fourth area for modifications of our theory concerns the potential for the substitution of ambulatory care for hospital-based services in closed-panel HMOs. Actually, our modifications in this area might be more appropriately identified as refinements; the results suggest that a more precise specification of the relationships may be anticipated. Because the proportion of the medical practice that involves prepaid patients is greatest in Kaiser model and non-Kaiser group model HMOs, we expect that future studies will find that substitution of ambulatory for hospital-based care is greatest in these two closed-panel types of HMOs. The reason for this should be clear. It is in the Kaiser model and non-Kaiser group model HMOs that physicians are most likely to be sensitive to the fiscal incentives of prepaid reimbursement structures because of their considerable proprietary interest in and dependence on the prepaid group practice's survival. Accordingly, we expect the substitution effect to be most marked in Kaiser model HMOs; it should also be clearly evident in non-Kaiser group model HMOs, although there the effect may not be so great. In both the staff model and IPA model HMO settings, however, we do not expect significant substitution effects because of the lack of a clear proprietary interest by staff model HMO physicians and because of the minimal participation in and therefore risk of IPA model HMO physicians in the prepaid practice. Thus, we expect that future studies of the relationship between the organization of medical practice and the substitution of ambulatory care for hospital-based services will focus primarily on identifying these effects in Kaiser and non-Kaiser group model HMOs.

Last are the modifications of our theoretical perspective concerning physicians' net incomes. The results of the hierarchical modeling of physicians' net incomes provided considerable support for our theory at the general level, inasmuch as several of the practice setting characteristics produced statistically significant effects. Although some of these effects were consistent with our theoretical expectations, others were not. On the one hand, the results showed that non-Kaiser group model and staff model HMO physicians had significantly lower net incomes than their group fee-for-service counterparts, or, for that matter, than their counterparts in IPA model HMOs or in solo fee-for-service practices. On the other hand, although not statistically significant at the .05 level (but at the .058 level), the regression coefficient for physicians in Kaiser model HMOs indicated that their net incomes were considerably higher than those of their counterparts in group fee-for-service practices or any of the other four practice settings. Although the lower income observed for physicians in non-Kaiser group model and staff model HMOs is consistent with our expectations, the nearly significantly higher net income of physicians in Kaiser model HMOs contradicts those expectations.

There is, however, an alternative explanation of these apparently contradictory findings. Among the three closed-panel types of HMOs (Kaiser model, non-Kaiser group model, and staff model), the Kaiser model HMOs are most stable, developed, and mature. For example, no Kaiser model HMO has ever filed for chapter 11 bankruptcy, nor has any been in serious financial straits. Kaiser model HMOs also enjoy the longest history of any form of prepaid group medical practice and are traditionally built upon strong, viable, existing medical groups in which all of the participant physicians have clear proprietary and career interests.

In contrast, physicians in staff model HMOs typically have no proprietary interests in the group itself and are often just beginning or ending their medical careers by affiliating with the staff model HMO. As a result, these physicians are not as likely to practice medicine in a profit-maximizing way because they are less likely to share in any profits that accrue. For two slightly different reasons, physicians in non-Kaiser group model HMOs (i.e., hybrid group model HMOs) may also be less likely to receive incomes comparable to those of their Kaiser model HMO counterparts. First, many of the new hybrid non-Kaiser group model HMOs have been formed to enhance the marketability of what had previously been basically group fee-for-service practices. Thus, many group practices have been motivated to become hybrid non-Kaiser group model HMOs to bolster economically weak medical practices. Second, their appearance is a recent development. There is no well-established tradition allowing the prepaid incentive structure to govern the practice of medicine for the prepaid patients, not to mention the nonprepaid patients.

This discussion suggests the following revision of our theoretical expectations. Physicians who participate in staff model HMOs appear to be at a turning point, usually at the beginning or the end of their careers. As a result, it would seem reasonable to expect the net incomes of physicians in staff model HMOs to be lower, perhaps significantly so, than those in either solo or group fee-for-service practice settings. Similarly, it would also seem reasonable to expect that net incomes for physicians in developing non-Kaiser group model (i.e., hybrid) HMOs would be lower than those in more developed and stable solo or group fee-for-service practices. For physicians in the more established and successful Kaiser model HMOs, however, it would seem reasonable that incomes may actually be greater than those of their counterparts in either solo or group fee-for-service practices. Accordingly, we would expect that future studies of the relationship between the organization of medical practice and physicians' net incomes will find the highest income levels among physicians in Kaiser model HMOs, followed by a cluster of nearly equivalent incomes of physicians in either solo or group fee-for-service practices or in IPA model HMOs, with the lowest income levels observed for physicians in staff model and non-Kaiser group model HMOs.

Policy Implications

Both our theory and our findings raise important considerations for the American health care delivery system. Two major policy implications deserve special attention. The first focuses on the general nature of structural alterations of the health care delivery system that might achieve cost containment and maintain quality health care. The second concerns a particularly popular approach to altering the structure of the health care delivery system; our research suggests it is not likely to succeed. We shall address each of these issues in turn.

If our research has demonstrated anything, it is that the organization of medical practice does, indeed, affect the practice of medicine. Moreover, these effects are logical, easily anticipated, and readily manipulated. As a result, it would seem most appropriate that policies designed to modify the present health care delivery system should manipulate the organizational incentive structures assessed herein.

This conclusion, of course, is not surprising. Indeed, Congress formally recognized the importance of the organization of medical practice in the practice of medicine in 1974 when it enacted the National Health Planning and Resources Development Act (PL 93–641). One of the most important dimensions of PL 93–641 was the establishment of ten specific national priorities for remedying the health care delivery system. Four of these ten focused on encouraging the development of new organizational forms of medical practice that were thought to facilitate cost containment while maintaining high quality health care. These four priorities addressed the development of vertically integrated alternative health care delivery systems, such as HMOs, which have the capacity to provide various levels of health care from the same site, in an organizational setting conducive to cost containment and quality health care. Initially, these ten national priorities were to be used as guidelines in the development of a national policy on health care and health care delivery (Warner 1977).

Consistent with this rudimentary national health care policy, several programs were instituted and special benefits were made available to stimulate the growth and development of multi-institutional systems, especially HMOs. The emphasis on HMOs reflected the general consensus that the principal culprits in the war of cost containment were the perverse fiscal incentives of the fee-for-service physician reimbursement system and the lack of peer regulation among physicians who traditionally practiced in solo settings. Closed-panel HMOs were thought to address both of these issues simultaneously, and thus seemed the most viable organizational intervention. As a result, the stage was set for massive federal fiscal and promotional support for the HMO concept.

The reader will note that as of the publication of this book, 11 years have passed since the National Health Planning and Resources Development Act of 1974 went into effect. Nonetheless, the tandem issues of cost containment and maintenance of high quality health care have yet to be resolved. Writing in a recent special issue of the *Milbank Memorial Fund Quarterly* devoted to the future financing of Medicare, Hadley (1984) addressed the key issues involved in considering alternative methods of paying physicians. Although specifically targeted to the issues involving paying physicians under Medicare, Hadley's remarks are most appropriate for our discussion of the general policy implications of the relationship between the organization of medical practice and the practice of medicine.

Hadley mentioned briefly the allegedly nonviable option of placing all physicians on a straight salary, as in the Veterans Administration system or the British National Health Service. He then discussed in detail three broad groups of alternative proposals designed to change physicians' practice arrangements, the unit of output Medicare pays for, and how Medicare determines the price it will pay for each service. Of principal interest to the present discussion is the review of the proposals designed to change physicians' practice arrangements. According to Hadley (1984, 284), this group of proposals includes

> a heterogeneous assortment of strategies, such as the health maintenance organization (HMO), the independent practice association (IPA), competitive bidding, the preferred provider organization (PPO), case management, health care brokers, and the primary care network. HMOs and IPAs are the most prevalent alternatives actually in existence, though they cover barely more than 5 percent of the nonelderly and an even smaller proportion of Medicare beneficiaries. The other alternatives are still experimental, with small-scale trials underway in a few places around the country.

Thus, although there are a number of strategies for changing physicians' practice arrangements in order to achieve cost containment, and although each of these strategies has in one way or another enjoyed preferential tax or regulatory treatment, they have neither individually nor collectively resulted in an appreciable reconfiguration and redirection of the American health care delivery system.

Although no two of these proposals are identical, they all rely upon one crucial operational incentive. According to Hadley (1984, 284):

> To varying degrees, these plans aim to change physician-practice arrangements, from independent fee-for-service practice to other organizational arrangements that increase physicians' incentives to monitor each other's behavior.

Indeed, all of these proposals are designed to replace the incentives of fee-for-service reimbursement with prepaid or capitation-based reimbursement mechanisms, and to increase the probability for peer regulation among physicians by creating incentives for them to practice in more bureaucratic as opposed to autonomous settings. By addressing these two key issues (reimbursement incentives and the probability of peer regulation), it was assumed that cost containment could be achieved while quality health care was maintained.

Unfortunately, the issue is not that simple, as Hadley (1984, 286–87) points out:

> These plans are not designed to be fiscally neutral. On the contrary, one of their key features is that they create financial conflicts between providers and patients. Limiting how much can be spent, and tying physicians' remuneration to how much they stay below the limit, creates incentives not to accept for treatment beneficiaries

who require more intensive care, and tilts the quality-cost and access-cost tradeoffs in favor of lower cost, quality, and access (i.e., to "cream-skim"). For those who believe that the current system favors too much quality and too much access, the lack of fiscal neutrality may be viewed as a plus. It should be recognized, though, that this would be a fundamental shift away from the traditional physician-patient relationship based on trust and agency.

Thus, Hadley identifies the ethical and moral dilemma of how to balance the perverse and opposite fiscal incentives facing physicians and patients. Initially it may have been naively assumed that the physician's fiscal incentive to both "skim" and "underprovide" in the prepaid setting would be equally offset by the incentive of the patient to "overuse" and "abuse" health care privileges. There is, however, no available evidence to demonstrate that these two incentives are, in fact, equally offsetting. That poses significant problems for the health care delivery system. On the one hand, if the perverse fiscal incentive facing physicians is stronger than that facing patients, then there will be a general underprovision of needed medical care in prepaid practice settings, and the more needy will be more likely to be prevented from participating in prepaid health care delivery systems. On the other hand, if the perverse patient's fiscal incentive is stronger than the physician's, then more health services will be consumed than are necessary. The former issue questions the very integrity of medicine as we now know it in the United States, while the latter prevents the achievement of cost containment.

Despite the conflicting incentives of patients and physicians in prepaid health care delivery systems, Hadley (1984, 287) favors the continued encouragement and development of these and other practice arrangements as competing alternatives to, but not substitutes for, fee-for-service practice settings. His reasoning is based on the assumption that although HMOs, PPOs, IPAs, and other prepaid alternative delivery systems will not become the mainstream of the American health care industry, they are likely to place increased pressures on fee-for-service practices. These pressures should, in turn, help to restrain both fee and expenditure growth in the future.

We agree with Hadley (1984) on two counts. First, prepaid health care delivery systems, especially HMOs, are not likely to gain a dominant market share in the United States in general, nor in more than a handful of isolated areas in particular. Second, despite their apparent inability to take over the health care market, HMOs and other alternative prepaid health care delivery systems will continue to provide competition for fee-for-service practices sufficient to result in increased pressures for cost containment.

We disagree, however, with Hadley's (1984) and others' focus on the overall organization of the medical practice setting as opposed to isolating the incentive bundles which compose that setting. In particular, our research clearly underscores two points: (1) the difference between prepaid and fee-for-service reimbursement mechanisms does affect the practice of medicine, and (2) certain organizational arrangements (i.e., more bureaucratic practice settings) facilitate cost containment (through greater inducements for peer review). Accordingly, instead of supporting any particular existing or new alternative health care delivery system, we implore policy makers to recognize that these two particular incentive structures produce the allegedly desired effects on the practice of medicine. Therefore, we urge policy makers not to nearsightedly focus on the particular form of an alternative health care delivery system, but to farsightedly focus on the use of the individual incentives that have been shown to produce the desired effects on the practice of medicine.

We would also point out that at the time Hadley (1984) wrote his provocative article, there were no major or definitive empirical assessments of the relationship between the organization of medical practice and the practice of medicine. Although our study is clearly not definitive, we believe that the results presented herein suggest that Hadley may have seriously underestimated the impact of the organization of medical practice on the practice of medicine.

The second policy issue that we wish to address concerns the implications of both our theory and our results for the viability of preferred provider organizations (PPOs). PPOs are one of the newest proposals to change practice arrangements in order to achieve cost containment while maintaining high quality health care (Federation of American Hospitals 1982). It would seem reasonable to begin with a clear understanding of what a PPO actually is. Unfortunately, there is no generally accepted definition of PPOs available at the present time (Ellwein 1982; Kodner 1982; Lundy and Blacker 1983; Mitlyng 1983). Simply stated, PPOs are groups of hospitals and physicians which contract on a fee-for-service basis with employers, insurance carriers, or third-party administrators to provide comprehensive medical service to subscribers (i.e., patients). If patients use the preferred providers, then they receive an economic incentive, usually in the form of no out-of-pocket costs (i.e., no deductibles or co-payments). Patients may, however, choose whomever they want as a provider; if they go outside of the preferred provider list, however, then they must pay the usual co-payments or deductibles. Employer groups who contract with the PPO usually receive discounts and other incentives that make offering the PPO cheaper than offering their existing insurance plans.

The following list of the five apparently common characteristics may help to clarify what PPOs are and are not (see Ellwein 1982):

— Provider panel
— Negotiated fee schedule
— Utilization and claims review system
— Consumer choice
— Quick turnaround of provider claims

The *provider panel* consists of a limited number of physicians and hospitals. This is analogous to the list of participating providers in an IPA, or to the closed panel in the Kaiser or non-Kaiser group model HMO. The actual insurance contract is between the panel of providers and the employer group. The *negotiated fee schedule* frequently reflects discounts from the usual, customary, and reasonable (UCR) fee structures in the community. These discounts average about 15 percent to 20 percent for physicians' services, and from 5 percent to 20 percent for hospital-based services. This is the incentive that makes the PPO attractive to the employer group. The *utilization and claims reviews* provide the PPO the data necessary to identify "expensive" from "nonexpensive" physicians and hospitals. This represents the basic control function of the PPO. Indeed, it is the single mechanism with which the PPO ensures that it will be cost containing, by the selection and maintenance of only cost-containing providers for its panel. *Consumer choice* involves the fact that patients need not choose providers only from the preferred panel. To encourage their use of the panel, however, patients usually receive a waiver of all out-of-pocket costs if they pick a provider from the panel. If patients do not use a provider from the preferred list, they are faced with about a 20 percent co-payment. This elimination of out-of-pocket costs is the incentive for the consumer to select the PPO. It is also indirectly one of the incentives for providers, inasmuch as it directs new patients their way; these new patients, of course, are insured and do not pose risks for nonpayment. The *quick turn around of provider claims* is perhaps the biggest incentive for providers, especially in terms of the enhanced cash flow associated with full payment, which often occurs in no more than 10 to 14 days.

What makes the PPO most attractive for patients is the choice of providers, PPO or otherwise, and the possibility of no out-of-pocket costs if they choose from the PPO panel. Moreover, PPO patients need not "lock in" to the PPO for the typical yearlong enrollment period like their counterparts in HMOs or Blue Cross/Blue Shield. Rather, PPO patients merely have a single policy that allows them to choose on a daily basis between PPO and non-PPO panel providers. Thus, they can retain their contacts with providers not on the PPO panel (at a cost of about a 20 percent co-payment) or use PPO panel provider specialists and hospitals as the need arises (with no out-of-pocket cost). In essence, it is the best of both worlds from the patient's perspective, at least theoretically.

From the physician's perspective, the PPO extracts a negotiated price that is lower than current UCR levels. In return, the PPO offers three offsetting incentives: (1) rapid turnaround on claims, (2) the potential for easy enlargement of the patient base, and (3) minimal financial risk, because the physician (or hospital) does not underwrite or guarantee the financial viability of the PPO. Moreover, the PPO concept allows the maintenance of the traditional fee-for-service system, albeit in a slightly modified form. Thus, the PPO might seem rather attractive from the physician's perspective as well.

Despite its apparent attractiveness to patients and physicians (as well as to hospitals), there are several reasons why we do not consider PPOs a viable method for obtaining significant cost containment while maintaining the quality of health care provided. First, there is no evidence to demonstrate that PPOs deliver cost containment in either the short run or the long run. (To be sure, it is not even clear how many PPOs there are, because there is no consensus on what a PPO is.) In this regard, the state of the art of evaluating PPOs today is remarkably similar to that of HMOs about a decade ago. The reader will recall that this was a period of time in the history of HMOs when policy makers simply took the promise of HMOs as gospel, in the absence of any solid evidence on performance. As we have seen, HMOs have not turned out to be the answer for resolving the crisis in the health care delivery system. We do not believe that PPOs will become that answer either.

The second reason that we do not consider PPOs to be a viable alternative health care delivery system involves the method by which physicians are reimbursed. The PPO relies on the fee-for-service reimbursement system, which has been identified as one of the basic causes of the cost-containment problem. We agree that in a good PPO, at least in principle, overproviders (or too-costly providers) will be identified, chastised, and if they do not cease overproviding (or being too costly), dropped from the PPO panel. Although this is theoretically pleasing, it is essentially the same argument that was used to justify IPAs. If the research reported herein establishes nothing else, it has clearly demonstrated the fact that the practice of medicine in IPA model HMOs is no different from that in group fee-for-service practice settings. Thus, IPA model HMOs cannot be relied upon to make the practice of medicine more cost containing. Because in many ways PPOs are an extension of IPA model HMOs, it also seems unlikely that PPOs will ever become the answer to the cost-containment question. Indeed, the only real difference between PPOs and IPAs involves the enhanced moral hazard facing patients in PPOs, which is most likely to result in increased demand for health services and subsequently higher rather than lower health care costs.

Third, we do not feel that PPOs will resolve the cost-containment issue because of their potential long-term effects, which are likely to approximate those of HMOs, in that both operate on reducing costs at the margin. For example, a PPO hospital discounts its prices by, say, 10 percent to attract new patients (i.e., new employer groups). Assuming that the PPO hospital succeeds, non-PPO hospitals have to trim their rates in a competitive response. How do the PPO hospital, and subsequently the non-PPO hospitals, then respond? There is, of course, a limit to price-cutting behavior. As the PPO grows, PPO providers will no longer be as able to offer such large discounts as "loss leaders." Similarly, non-PPO competitors already face substantial price competition from, among others, HMOs, and they will no longer be as able to offer such large counterdiscounts. How much additional price cutting is currently possible is an open question. What is not questionable, however, is that eventually the health care delivery system will be so lean that it will not be possible to offset the systemwide costs of either increased demand or high general inflation by increased organizational efficiencies. Therefore, although the short-run price-discounting scheme of the PPO may seem attractive, especially to those providers who enter at the early stages of the movement, it holds little promise for either later entrants in particular or long-term stable results throughout the system in general.

The final reason that we are not enchanted with the prospects of PPOs' achieving cost containment is the way in which PPOs try to be cost containing. Three methods are discussed in the PPO literature: (1) effectively using discounts, which implies success by working at the margins, (2) bringing only "cost-conscious" providers into the system, and (3) employing rigorous utilization review and control mechanisms. The first approach, using discounts, is the easiest; it is what most PPOs rely on. We do not believe, however, that discounts can provide anything other than a short-term marketing incentive to capture employer groups. The second approach, careful selection, can very easily result in playing one physician against another, and a more fragmented, schismatized provider pool will not accomplish much (see Carlova 1983). It is in the utilization review and control mechanisms that the future lies. Indeed, that is what makes closed-panel HMOs (especially Kaiser and non-Kaiser group model HMOs) effective, and it could also make PPOs effective. Often dubbed "bureaucratic medicine," however, such review mechanisms are not attractive to most physicians. If they were, solo fee-for-service practice would not have dominated American medicine for so long. Perhaps, however, in this era of an increasing physician supply coupled with "medi-flation," the practice of quasi-bureaucratic medicine—that is, group practice without really having the group—will become attractive to more physicians. Even so, it may still fail to contain rising health care costs.

To obtain a more durable resolution of the problem of rising health care costs we must learn more about the connection between the organization of medical practice and the practice of medicine. Although our theoretical and empirical work have contributed toward an understanding of this relationship, much remains to be done. We need better measurement if our empirical models are to become more powerful. We need greater specification of the process by which organizational structure affects individual behavior if our theories are to become more useful in shaping health care policy. The theoretical interests of sociologists and economists are clearly intertwined with the practical concerns of the public and policymakers. It would appear, then, that the interests of both groups will be best served by their continued mutual pursuit of learning more about the organization of medical practice and the practice of medicine.

References

Berki, Sylvester, and Marie Ashcraft. 1980. "HMO enrollment: Who joins what and why: A review of the literature." *Milbank Memorial Fund Quarterly* 58:588–632.

Carlova, John. 1983. "How PPOs turn doctor against doctor." *Medical Economics* September 19:86–92.

Ellwein, Linda. 1982. "Preferred provider organizations: A new form of competitive health plan?" *Colorado Medicine* March: 1–2.

Federation of American Hospitals. 1982. "Health care industry, business show increasing interest in PPO concept." *Federation of American Hospitals Review* July:12–18.

Fink, Ray. 1980. "HMO physicians' recruitment stymied by higher fee-for-service salaries." *Group Health News* 21:8–9.

Freidson, Eliot. 1970. *Profession of Medicine: A Study of the Sociology of Applied Knowledge.* New York: Harper and Row.

Hadley, Jack. 1984. "How should Medicare pay physicians." *Milbank Memorial Fund Quarterly* 62:279–99.

Held, Phillip, and Uwe Reinhardt. 1979. *Analysis of Economic Performance in Medical Group Practices.* Princeton, N.J.: Mathematica Policy Research.

Kodner, Karen. 1982. "Competition: getting a fix on PPOs." *Hospitals* November 16:59–66.

Luft, Harold. 1978a. "How do health maintenance organizations achieve their savings? Rhetoric and evidence." *New England Journal of Medicine* 298:1336–43.

_____. 1978b. "Why do HMOs seem to provide more health maintenance services?" *Milbank Memorial Fund Quarterly* 56:140–68.

_____. 1980. "Trends in medical care costs: Do HMOs lower the rate of growth?" *Medical Care* 18:1–16.

_____. 1981. *Health Maintenance Organizations: Dimensions of Performance.* New York: Wiley.

_____. 1983. "Health maintenance organizations." In *Handbook of Health, Health Care, and the Health Professions,* edited by David Mechanic. New York: Free Press.

Lundy, Robert, and Richard Blacker. 1983. "Preferred provider organizations: The latest response to health care competition—an overview." *Healthcare Financial Management* July:14–18.

Mechanic, David. 1975. "The organization of medical practice and practice orientations among physicians in prepaid and nonprepaid primary care settings." *Medical Care* 13:189–204.

Mitlyng, Joseph. 1983. "PPOs: Implications for management." *Medical Group Management* September:38–47.

PL 93–641. 1974. *The National Health Planning and Resources Development Act of 1974.* Washington, D.C.: Government Printing Office.

Warner, Judith. 1977. "The National Health Planning and Resources Development Act of 1974." In the *Standard Medical Almanac.* Chicago: Marquis Academic Media.

Appendix:
Facsimile of
PSP-14 Questionnaire

PERIODIC SURVEY OF PHYSICIANS

CENTER FOR HEALTH SERVICES RESEARCH AND DEVELOPMENT

American Medical Association
535 North Dearborn Street
Chicago, Illinois 60610

© American Medical Association 1980

Dear Doctor:

In its efforts to obtain reliable information on the practice of medicine, the American Medical Association instituted the Periodic Survey of Physicians in 1966. Results from each survey have been published annually in the Profile of Medical Practice. The cooperation exhibited by the responding physicians demonstrates that the profession is willing to participate in the development of valid, reliable data on medical practice.

Your assistance is now being sought so that the series may be broadened to include both new information and larger segments of the profession. The results will enable the calculation of national, regional, and specialty averages with stated reliability. These surveys have been very useful in representing the physician's practice situation. All responses will be handled in the strictest confidence and only aggregate figures will be published.

The success of this survey and, therefore, its usefulness to the individual physician and to the profession depends on your reply. Your cooperation in this important project is greatly appreciated.

Sincerely,

James H. Sammons, M.D.
Executive Vice President

INSTRUCTIONS

Please answer ALL of the following questions. For questions which are NOT APPLICABLE to your practice, please mark N.A. For questions where the appropriate response is ZERO, please mark a ZERO rather than leaving the response blank or using a dash. If you do not have specific information, please provide an estimate. Please return your completed questionnaire in the enclosed envelope.

A. PRACTICE CHARACTERISTICS

1. Please give the SPECIALTY from which you derived 50% or more
of your 1979 MEDICAL income.. _____

2. How many weeks did you practice in 1979? (EXCLUDE residency, medical meetings,
military service, vacations and similar absences from practice.)........................ _____WEEKS

3. Is your practice organized as a professional corporation?   ☐ Yes   ☐ No

4. Which of the following best describes the size and type of your main practice arrangement?
   ☐ Solo (Individual, self-employed)

   ☐ Partnership or Group Practice. Please indicate the number of physicians INCLUDING yourself.. _____

   ☐ Other   _____
                                                (Please describe)

5. If you are in a partnership or group practice arrangement, which of the following BEST describes your method
of income distribution?   ☐ Equal distribution   ☐ Straight salary

   ☐ Salary plus share of profit   ☐ Fee-for-service (expense sharing)

   ☐ Other   _____
                                                 (Please describe)

B. HOURS PRACTICED AND PATIENT VISITS

1. How many TOTAL HOURS did you practice during your most recent COMPLETE WEEK
of practice? (EXCLUDE "on-call" hours not actually worked.)........................ _____HOURS

2. How many of these HOURS were spent in providing DIRECT PATIENT CARE or patient-related
service? (INCLUDE interpreting X-rays, lab tests, etc. EXCLUDE administrative
tasks, meetings, etc.).. _____HOURS

3. How many HOURS did you spend in the following activities during your most
recent COMPLETE WEEK of practice?

   a. Seeing patients in office... _____HOURS

   b. Seeing patients in hospital (inpatient, outpatient, etc.)....................... _____HOURS

   c. In business administration activities (employee supervision, filling out
   insurance forms, etc.)... _____HOURS

4. How many PATIENT VISITS did you have during your most recent COMPLETE WEEK of practice:

   a. At the office... _____VISITS

   b. At the hospital... _____VISITS

5. How many TOTAL PATIENT VISITS did you have during your most complete
week of practice.. _____VISITS

6. How many total patients do you currently have? _____

7. Please give the approximate time that a patient wishing to see you has to wait:

   a. To be scheduled for a routine office visit.

       A New Patient:_____DAYS   An Established Patient:_____DAYS

   b. To see you after arriving for a scheduled appointment:_____MINUTES

C. PRACTICE SETTINGS

1. How *important* was each of these issues to your *choice* of solo or group practice?

(Please check one box in each row)

	Very Important	Important	Not Important
a. Business side of medical practice	[]	[]	[]
b. Predictability of practice schedule	[]	[]	[]
c. Personal autonomy in delivering care	[]	[]	[]
d. Practice location	[]	[]	[]
e. Earnings potential	[]	[]	[]

2. Do you individually or through a group practice have a formal agreement or contract with an organization that provides prepaid health services (e.g., HMO, IPA, etc.)?   Yes []   No []

3. If yes, please indicate the name of this organization:

_____

Name of Organization   City   State   Zip

4. What percentage of your patients belong to this prepaid health organization: _____%

5. Please specify the name and location of the hospital to which you MOST FREQUENTLY admit patients. If you do not admit patients to a hospital, check this box [] and proceed to question 7.

_____

Name of Hospital   City   State   Zip

6. How many years have you had admitting privileges at this hospital? _____ YEARS

7. Are you a member of your local PSRO?   Yes   No

D. FEES AND REIMBURSEMENT

1. For each of the following procedures, please indicate your CURRENT USUAL FEE: (If you do not have a fee-for-service practice, please check this box [] and disregard this question.)

a. Office visit, NEW patient, brief evaluation, history, examination and/or treatment...................................$_____.00   N.A.

b. Office visit, ESTABLISHED patient, brief examination and/or treatment, same or new illness...................$_____.00   N.A.

c. Appendectomy...$_____.00   N.A.

d. Periodic or annual type examination, established patient adult, exclude lab, X-ray....................................$_____.00   N.A.

e. Hospital visit, new or established patient, brief examination, evaluation and/or treatment, same illness...............$_____.00   N.A.

2. Please estimate the percentage of your current patients whose principal HEALTH INSURANCE coverage for physician's services is:

   a. Medicare.. _____ %

   b. Medicaid.. _____ %

   c. Prepayment-Capitation (HMO, IPA)... _____ %

   d. Other health insurance plans (Blue Cross/Blue Shield, commercial plans, etc.)............... _____ %

   e. No health insurance.. _____ %

E. INCOMES AND EXPENSES

1. What were your total tax-deductible PROFESSIONAL EXPENSES in 1979. (If you shared expenses with other physicians, indicate your share only.)

   a. 1979 Professional Expenses $_____,000

   b. PROJECTED 1980 Professional Expenses $_____,000

2. What was your 1979 INDIVIDUAL NET INCOME BEFORE TAXES from medical practice? (INCLUDE all income from fees, salaries, retainers, etc., as well as the value of all fringe benefits paid on your behalf, e.g., Keogh Plan.)

   a. 1979 Individual Net Income Before Taxes $_____,000

   b. PROJECTED 1980 Individual Net Income Before Taxes $_____,000

3. Please list the single most expensive piece of medical equipment you purchased during the past five years:

Name of Equipment	Cost	Year

4. What were your total tax-deductible PROFESSIONAL EXPENSES for the following items in 1979? (If you shared expenses, indicate only your share.)

   a. Total non-physician payroll expenses (INCLUDING fringe benefits)................... $_____.00

   b. Professional liability (malpractice) insurance................................ $ .00

   c. Medical equipment expenses (annual depreciation, leases, rent)................... $_____.00

   d. Office expenses (mortgage, rent, utilities, etc.)................................ $_____.00

The physician code numbers printed at right are needed during the survey to relate information from this questionnaire to the biographical and educational characteristics of each respondent.

Please detach your name and address before returning this questionnaire.

Index of Authors

Index of Subjects

established patients, 82, 83, 87;
physician estimates of, 54, 55; physician estimates, validity of, 54;
scheduling, 64, 94, 143; by specialty,
83, 87, 91; waiting rooms, 89–93,
143

Referrals: patterns, 4–6; psychiatric, 16,
17; by setting, 16, 17, 23
Regression coefficients: expenses, 125;
hours worked in direct patient care,
110; hours worked, total, 109; income, 124; patient queues, 84–85,
90; patient visits, 116, 117; scheduling, 84–85; time spent with patients,
95, 96; waiting room, 90
Regression equation: coding algorithm,
78, 79; hierarchical modeling, 81, 82
Regulation, in HMO, 40
Reimbursement: cost-minus, 1; cost-plus,
1; incentives, 15, 147–51
Relationship, patient-practitioner, 28, 31,
34
Reliability of PSP-14, 52, 53, 141, 142
Responsibility, medical, 26

Sample, physician, 56, 57, 59
Sanctions, 4
Satisfaction, client, 20–22
Scheduling, established patients, 87–89;
effect of attitudinal characteristics, 89;
effect of environmental characteristics,
88; effect of practice setting, 89;
effect of sociodemographic characteristics, 87, 88; by specialty, 87, 88
Scheduling, new patients, 83–87; effect
of attitudinal characteristics, 86, 87;
effect of environmental characteristics,
83, 86; effect of practice setting, 87;
effect of sociodemographic characteristics, 83; by specialty, 83
Self-selection of physicians, 2, 11,
25–29, 33, 43, 68, 79, 80
Socialization, educational, 3
Sociodemographic characteristics: 76, 77,

83, 87, 88, 89, 91, 94, 97, 99, 108,
111, 113, 115, 118, 126, 127, 129
Sociodemographic characteristics, effects
on: expenses, 129; hospital visits,
120; hours worked, in patient care,
113; hours worked, total, 108, 111;
income, 126, 127; office visits, 115,
118; scheduling established patients,
87, 88; scheduling new patients, 83;
time spent per patient, in hospital,
99; time spent per patient, in office,
94, 97; waiting time, 89, 91
Sociodemographic characteristics,
measures of, 76, 77
Sociological influences, 22–24
Solo practice: fee-for-service, 4–7, 12;
versus group, 11–13
Specialty. *See* Medical specialty
Sponsorship, physician, 7
Surgery, reasons for exclusion from
analysis, 76

"Target-Time" hypothesis, 14, 15, 137
Task: delegation, 16; inventory, physician, 53, 54
Technology, adoption, 15
Theory modifications, 142–47; hospital
visit length, 144, 145; physician net
income, 146, 147; substitution of
ambulatory for hospital care, 146;
waiting room queues, 143, 144;
workload characteristics, 145
Time spent with patients, 80, 81,
93–101, 137, 139–140, 144, 145;
calculation method, 80, 81. *See also*
Workload
Time spent with patients, in hospital:
effect of attitudinal characteristics, 99,
100; effect of environmental characteristics, 99; effect of practice setting,
64, 100, 140; effect of sociodemographic characteristics, 99; by
specialty, 99
Time spent with patients, office: effect
of attitudinal characteristics, 98; effect

of environmental characteristics, 97, 98; effect of practice setting, 64, 98, 139, 140; effect of sociodemographic characteristics, 94, 97; by specialty, 97
Treatment, differences in, 23

Utilization: of ancillary services, 32, 33; and HMOs, 30–34; and organization, 23

Validity of PSP–14, 53–56, 141, 142
Veterans Administration, 149

Waiting time, 89–93; effect of attitudinal characteristics, 91, 92; effect of environmental characteristics, 91; effect of practice setting, 92; effect of sociodemographic characteristics, 89, 91; by specialty, 91

Western United States, 77, 78, 83, 86, 88, 91, 97, 99, 111, 113, 118, 121, 127, 129, 130
Workload, 105–23, 137, 138, 140, 145; measures of, 107. *See also* Time spent with patients
Workload, direct patient care, 106, 112–14, 137, 138, 140, 145; effect of attitudinal characteristics, 114; effect of environmental characteristics, 113, 114; effect of practice setting, 114, 137, 138, 140, 145; effect of sociodemographic characteristics, 113; by specialty, 113
Workload, total hours, 60, 106, 108–12, 137, 138, 140, 145; effect of attitudinal characteristics, 111, 112; effect of environmental characteristics, 111; effect of practice setting, 60, 112, 137, 138, 140, 145; effect of sociodemographic characteristics, 108, 111; by specialty, 111

About the Authors

FREDRIC D. WOLINSKY received his Ph.D. in sociology from Southern Illinois University at Carbondale in 1977. He has been assistant professor of sociology at East Carolina University, senior research associate at the Center for Health Services Research and Development at the American Medical Association, and associate professor and director of health services research at St. Louis University Medical Center. Dr. Wolinsky now holds a senior-level faculty appointment in the department of sociology at Texas A&M University. There he continues to study the health and illness behavior of the elderly, with the support of a Research Career Development Award from the National Institute on Aging. Among Dr. Wolinsky's many publications is *The Sociology of Health: Principles, Professions, and Issues* (Little, Brown 1980), as well as more than 30 articles in refereed journals, including *Health Services Research*, the *American Journal of Public Health*, the *Journal of Health and Social Behavior*, *Medical Care*, *Inquiry*, *Social Science and Medicine*, the *Milbank Memorial Fund Quarterly*, the *Journal of Gerontology*, and *The Gerontologist*, among others.

WILLIAM D. MARDER is a Ph.D. candidate in economics at the University of Chicago. Formerly assistant professor of economics at Roosevelt University, Mr. Marder joined the Center for Health Services Research and Development (now the Center for Health Policy Research) at the American Medical Association in 1980 as research associate. In 1983 Mr. Marder was promoted to senior economist, and in 1985 he became director, department of health resource analysis. Mr. Marder has published a number of articles in both economic and health services research journals, including the *American Journal of Public Health*, the *Journal of Human Resources*, *Medical Care*, the *Journal of Medical Education*, and *Medical Group Management*.

About the Authors

FREDRIC D. WOLINSKY received his Ph.D. in sociology from Southern Illinois University at Carbondale in 1977. He has been assistant professor of sociology at East Carolina University, senior research associate at the Center for Health Services Research and Development at the American Medical Association, and associate professor and director of health services research at St. Louis University Medical Center. Dr. Wolinsky now holds a senior-level faculty appointment in the department of sociology at Texas A&M University. There he continues to study the health and illness behavior of the elderly, with the support of a Research Career Development Award from the National Institute on Aging. Among Dr. Wolinsky's many publications is *The Sociology of Health: Principles, Professions, and Issues* (Little, Brown 1980), as well as more than 30 articles in refereed journals, including *Health Services Research*, the *American Journal of Public Health*, the *Journal of Health and Social Behavior*, *Medical Care*, *Inquiry*, *Social Science and Medicine*, the *Milbank Memorial Fund Quarterly*, the *Journal of Gerontology*, and *The Gerontologist*, among others.

WILLIAM D. MARDER is a Ph.D. candidate in economics at the University of Chicago. Formerly assistant professor of economics at Roosevelt University, Mr. Marder joined the Center for Health Services Research and Development (now the Center for Health Policy Research) at the American Medical Association in 1980 as research associate. In 1983 Mr. Marder was promoted to senior economist, and in 1985 he became director, department of health resource analysis. Mr. Marder has published a number of articles in both economic and health services research journals, including the *American Journal of Public Health*, the *Journal of Human Resources*, *Medical Care*, the *Journal of Medical Education*, and *Medical Group Management*.